The Nurse Professional

Deborah Dolan Hunt, PhD, MS, RN, is an associate professor of nursing at the College of New Rochelle. She has spent most of her career in nursing education, initially in staff development and currently in an academic setting. She began her nursing career in critical care and has held several leadership positions. She is the cofounder and codirector of the Nurse Advocacy Forum at the College of New Rochelle. This forum was developed to offer mentoring, support, advocacy, and networking opportunities to nursing students and new graduate nurses as they transition into professional practice. She is currently serving as one of the coleads for the New York State Future of Nursing's Action Coalition in the Northern Metropolitan Region. She is a member of the advisory board for the Advance Healthcare Network. She is a member of Community Board #10 in the Bronx and the chairperson of its Health and Human Services Committee. Dr. Hunt is a fellow of the New York Academy of Medicine and an ambassador for the Patient Centered Outcomes Research Institute. She is a member of Sigma Theta Tau International Honor Society of Nursing and received the Zeta Omega research award for her doctoral dissertation and was the Sigma Theta Tau Zeta Omega Scholar from 2010 to 2011. Her doctoral dissertation was titled "Nurses' and Supervisors' Value Congruence, Leadership Support and Patient Outcomes and the Effect on Job Satisfaction and Intent to Leave" and her research has been published in the *Journal of Nursing Management*. Her research interests are in nursing turnover, job satisfaction, leadership, patient outcomes, and new-nurse transition. Dr. Hunt is the author of *The New Nurse Educator* (Springer, 2013). She has published multiple articles and has presented locally, nationally, and globally. She holds a PhD from Adelphi University, an MS degree in Nursing Administration from the College of New Rochelle, and a BSN from Mercy College.

The Nurse Professional

Leveraging Your Education for Transition Into Practice

Deborah Dolan Hunt , PhD, MS, RN

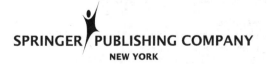

SPRINGER PUBLISHING COMPANY
NEW YORK

Springer Publishing Company, LLC
11 West 42nd Street
New York, NY 10036
www.springerpub.com

Acquisitions Editor: Margaret Zuccarini
Production Editor: Kris Parrish
Composition: Integra Software Services Pvt. Ltd.

ISBN: 978-0-8261-6877-1
e-book ISBN: 978-0-8261-6878-8
Instructor's Materials ISBN: 978-0-8261-7163-4

Instructor's Materials: Qualified instructors may request supplements by emailing textbook@springerpub.com

14 15 16 17 / 5 4 3 2 1

The author and the publisher of this Work have made every effort to use sources believed to be reliable to provide information that is accurate and compatible with the standards generally accepted at the time of publication. Because medical science is continually advancing, our knowledge base continues to expand. Therefore, as new information becomes available, changes in procedures become necessary. We recommend that the reader always consult current research and specific institutional policies before performing any clinical procedure. The author and publisher shall not be liable for any special, consequential, or exemplary damages resulting, in whole or in part, from the readers' use of, or reliance on, the information contained in this book. The publisher has no responsibility for the persistence or accuracy of URLs for external or third-party Internet websites referred to in this publication and does not guarantee that any content on such websites is, or will remain, accurate or appropriate.

Library of Congress Cataloging-in-Publication Data

Hunt, Deborah Dolan, author.
 The nurse professional : leveraging your education for transition into practice / Deborah Dolan Hunt.
    p. ; cm.
 Includes bibliographical references and index.
 ISBN 978-0-8261-6877-1—ISBN 978-0-8261-6878-8 (e-book)
 I. Title.
 [DNLM: 1. Nurse's Role. 2. Education, Nursing. 3. Vocational Guidance. WY 87]
 RT82
 610.7306′9--dc23

                                                                  2014032182

Special discounts on bulk quantities of our books are available to corporations, professional associations, pharmaceutical companies, health care organizations, and other qualifying groups. If you are interested in a custom book, including chapters from more than one of our titles, we can provide that service as well.

For details, please contact:
Special Sales Department, Springer Publishing Company, LLC
11 West 42nd Street, 15th Floor, New York, NY 10036-8002
Phone: 877-687-7476 or 212-431-4370; Fax: 212-941-7842
E-mail: sales@springerpub.com

This book is dedicated to all nursing students and nurses—past, present, and future—and, of course, to my family—Pat and Rita Dolan; Maureen Dolan; my husband, Brian; my children, Brian, Meaghan, and John; as well as all the Dolans, the Tenetys, and the Hunts—and to my friends, especially my friend and mentor, Dr. Connie Vance; Dr. Jane White; and my friends and colleagues at the College of New Rochelle, Adelphi University, and Montefiore Medical Center. And, last but not least, to our foundress: Florence Nightingale.

Contents

Foreword

This is an important book at this particular point in time because of the health care reform initiatives taking place both nationally and internationally. These initiatives position nurses for the assumption of leadership roles in increasing access to quality health care, particularly for vulnerable populations. To assume their rightful roles as well as new positions of leadership that reflect the evolving landscape of health care, and to assume these roles effectively upon graduation, nurses must pay attention to their transition from student to professional, including the transition into leadership roles.

Transition theory, one of the effective frameworks discussed in this book, provides insight into the experiences, responses, and various outcomes of the transition from student to professional and from professional nursing to leadership roles. New graduates, in particular, experience the confusion that results from unfamiliar environments, the uncertainty of facing the unknown, the vulnerability of disconnectedness from support systems, and the disruption associated with lack of confidence in performing new sets of behaviors or performing known behaviors in new environments. These experiences may render new graduates ineffective, inefficient, or unsatisfied and may lead to attrition or burnout. Time and prolonged experience alone may help new graduates in developing confidence, mastery in providing care, and expertise in clinical judgments, as well as in the acquisition of supportive colleagues and environments. However, a more effective, proactive approach is the use of a more systematic, deliberate set of strategies to enhance the effectiveness of new graduates' well-being, as well as the well-being of the organizations in which they work.

This book provides a solid foundation for the development of programs that ensure the academic and professional success of new graduates during and at the completion of their transitions using the concepts from transition theory (Meleis, in press), as well as other theories. This requires clarity on roles, competencies, and meanings; the support of mentors and coaches, role models, and preceptors; opportunities for dialogue and debriefings about the meaning of experiences; mobilization of support systems; and research strategies to enhance healthy transitions. One important variable in achieving effectiveness is the identification of critical points and milestones for the delivery of each strategy. This book provides all of that and more, supporting each strategy and proposed action with theoretical and research evidence. It includes theories that inform and explain experiences and responses, personal and environmental changes, and tools to use, supported by advice on ways by which nurses can position themselves for leadership positions. Becoming a leader is one outcome of a transition that is well experienced and well supported.

By addressing self-care, ethical, and moral issues, as well as the process for securing first positions and assuring preparedness for subsequent positions and leadership roles, Dr. Deborah Hunt provides a full background on the definition, scope, and domain of the discipline of nursing and its properties of health, well-being, and attention to the environment, along with a focus on interactions and collaboration. In this book, she effectively provides a model for how different components, concepts, and properties of the domain of nursing may be connected.

Although this book is focused on nurses' experiences with their own transitions, it also provides the knowledge base that nurses can use when caring for clients who are experiencing their own transitions, such as transitions of becoming first-time mothers or fathers, of patients in or out of hospitals, or of the elderly who are in or out of rehabilitation facilities. Because nurses deal with patients in transition on a daily basis, they will find this book useful in providing the knowledge needed to make these transitions healthy, effective, and productive. The outcomes that Dr. Hunt strives for in the transition of new graduates are similar to other transition outcomes. These include developing a sense of mastery, becoming resourceful, engaging in healthy interactions, and experiencing a sense of well-being and integrated identity. Healthy transitions affect the health of organizations and ultimately the quality of care they provide, the health of the team with whom they work, the collaborations that are forged, and the partnerships that are developed. This book provides the foundation that will ultimately lead to more effective roles for nurses in shaping the structure of care as well as the nature of care provided.

This book should be reviewed and used by those who are anticipating or experiencing changes in their roles and positions, preparing graduates for their professional roles, or employing and launching graduates into professional roles. It supports the assertion that the discipline of nursing is about the science and art of transitions.

Afaf I. Meleis, PhD, DrPS (hon), FAAN
Dean Emerita, School of Nursing
Professor of Nursing and Sociology
University of Pennsylvania
School of Nursing
Philadelphia, Pennsylvania

REFERENCES

Meleis, A.I. (2010). *Transitions theory: Middle range and situation specific theories in research and practice*. New York, NY: Springer Publishing Company.

Meleis, A.I. (in press). Transitions. In M. E. Parker & M. Smith (Eds.), *Nursing theories and nursing practice* (4th ed.). Philadelphia, PA: F. A. Davis Company.

Preface

The more that you read, the more things you will know. The more that you learn, the more places you'll go.

—Dr. Seuss

This book is a culmination of my life's work as a nurse, educator, and researcher. I still remember my own transition—the excitement, the challenges, the tears, and the triumphs. Throughout the years I have met many nurses who have shared similar experiences; thankfully, many of them overcame the challenges, but unfortunately, some of them were so disillusioned they left their positions and, in some cases, the profession. It is my hope that this book and the continued research on new-nurse transition will in the future change the transition experience for new nurses around the world.

I spent a good portion of my professional career in staff development and was responsible for recruiting and orientating both new and experienced nurses. Often, there was a high turnover rate that related to a difficult transition period or a poor fit between the nurse and the work environment. This prompted me to explore nursing turnover, job satisfaction, and new-nurse transition. In fact, my doctoral dissertation focused on nursing job satisfaction and anticipated turnover, with one of the major themes being leadership support.

When I moved to academia, I experienced new-nurse transition from a different perspective, and in response to students' challenges, developed the College of New Rochelle's Nurse Advocacy Forum with my colleague, friend, and mentor, Dr. Connie Vance. The purpose of this forum is to offer advocacy, support, networking, professional development, leadership, and mentoring to students and new graduate nurses. Developing and researching new-nurse transition for the Nurse

Advocacy Forum, in addition to my past experiences and research, have helped me gain a better understanding of the needs of the new nurse that is the impetus for this book. I have come to understand the significance of the foundations laid and experiences gained through-out nursing school, and the need for continued support and knowledge development throughout the transition into professional practice. Some of the themes that new nurses identified as challenges during the Nurse Advocacy Forum meetings were:

- Insecurity about clinical knowledge and lack of self-confidence
- Importance of peer support—"leaning on each other"—and mentors
- Lack of support
- Importance of time management and organizational skills
- "Reality shock," "bullying"
- Work satisfaction/dissatisfaction and turnover intent
- Importance of self-care, advocacy, and networking
- Issues with communication and delegation

As you read this book you will learn about the many different issues and factors that inform your practice and strategies for overcoming the challenges you will face. The foundational development achieved during nursing school has a significant impact on your transition into professional practice; this book provides you with invaluable advice and strategies for continued success as your career progresses.

This book is divided into four major parts. Part I includes the first six chapters and provides an overview of the nursing profession and the significance of academic success in your nursing program. Strategies for success include good study habits, engaging in self-care activities, and learning how to advocate. The importance of portfolio development, understanding the Quality and Safety Education for Nurses (QSEN) competencies, and patient safety issues are also reviewed. An overview of the legal, moral, and ethical issues that inform your role as a student and nurse is provided in Chapter 6.

Part II focuses on the path from graduation to National Council Licensure Examination for Registered Nurses (NCLEX-RN®) success and your first nursing position. You will learn strategies for passing your exam and how to develop a résumé, cover letter, and interview skills necessary to gain a position.

Part III provides a more in-depth review of the issues relating to transition into professional practice and covers transition theory and transition process as well as strategies to guide you through this experience. In addition to learning about the role of the nurse generalist and the importance of time management and organization, you will develop skills to aid in delegation, leadership, and clinical practice. You will also learn techniques for dealing with bullying and all forms of disruptive behavior.

Part IV focuses on continuing role development and your continuing transition, with an emphasis on the importance of developing goals and objectives along with a 5-year plan to guide you through your journey into professional practice.

Material to accompany this book's content for qualified instructors is available from Springer Publishing Company by e-mailing *textbook@springerpub.com.*

This is an exciting time in nursing and health care, and as a student and new nurse you need to keep abreast of the current and future state of nursing and health care. In accordance with the Institute of Medicine's (IOM) *The Future of Nursing* report, you must commit to being a lifelong learner and be well versed in the current research, policies, regulations, and agencies that govern and inform health care and the profession of nursing.

The transition from student to registered professional nurse is filled with challenges and rewards and it is my hope that you will find this book helpful as you complete your academic program and transition into your professional practice role. I also hope that you will experience the same joy and passions that I have had through my tenure as a nurse, educator, leader, and scholar.

Deborah Dolan Hunt

PART I

Foundations for Success

CHAPTER 1

Introduction and Overview—World of Professional Nursing

Don't limit yourself. Many people limit themselves to what they think they can do. You can go as far as your mind lets you. What you believe, you can achieve.

—Mary Kay Ash

OBJECTIVES

After reading this chapter, the reader will be able to:

- Understand the role of the nurse generalist
- Discuss licensure and accreditation organizations that inform nursing practice
- Understand the Nurse Practice Act and the American Nurses Association (ANA) Code of Ethics
- Discuss the National Council of State Boards of Nursing (NCSBN) —Transition into Practice Model
- Discuss the role of the NCSBN in National Council Licensure Examinations (NCLEX)-RN®
- Identify key components of the Institute of Medicine (IOM) *Future of Nursing* report
- Understand the different career paths nursing can follow

Welcome to the world of nursing. You are well on your way to a most rewarding and exciting career. In addition to your formal program of study, there is much to learn about your profession and the information contained in this book helps guide you through your experiences as a student nurse and as a new graduate as you transition into your professional practice role.

This chapter provides a historical overview of nursing education and professional nursing practice from the days of Florence Nightingale to current-day practice. Although many programs do not offer a specific course on the history of nursing, many include it in the foundational nursing courses. Interestingly, some scholars are advocating for its formal inclusion in all nursing curricula. Our history is rich with nurses such as Florence Nightingale, "foundress of modern nursing"; Mary Seacole, a Jamaican nurse during the Crimean war; Clara Barton, a Civil War nurse who founded the American Red Cross; Virginia Henderson, who has been described as the "foremost nurse of the 20th century"; Jean Watson, who is a renowned nursing theorist; and Patricia Benner, who is a well-known scholar and theorist. These are just a small example of the nurses who embarked on a path because they cared about health and wellness, and the profession of nursing. You are now joining the ranks of these amazing and inspirational nurses and will add to the richness of our profession in your own unique way. As you go along your path, always believe in yourself, and know that nursing chose you just as much as you chose nursing.

Nursing education programs, whether associate degree, diploma, or baccalaureate degree, prepare students to become nurse generalists. After graduation and successful licensure, nurses transition into their professional practice role. During this transition nurses will most often select a specialty area. Some nurses stay in their specialty area for their entire career, whereas others work in several specialty areas before they find their niche. Nursing practice is guided by legal and accrediting bodies. It is also informed by theory, ethics, and moral codes. Therefore, it is important for all nurses to be knowledgeable about the factors that inform their professional practice. This chapter will also contain information about the role of national and state education boards and the National Council of State Boards of Nursing Transition into Practice model. Because of its impact on the nursing profession, the IOM's report on *The Future of Nursing* will also be included in this chapter. It is vital for all nurses to be knowledgeable about the many factors that influence health care and the nursing profession. There are many career options available to registered professional nurses and you may be surprised at some of the exciting roles you may aspire to after you graduate.

HISTORICAL OVERVIEW

The nursing profession and the role of nurses have undergone many changes since the days of Florence Nightingale. However, the underpinnings and foundations remain somewhat consistent. Indeed, Florence Nightingale is considered the founder of modern nursing, and is credited with being the first nurse to conduct research and to use what we refer to today as evidenced-based practice in her care of the sick and the wounded. She is also credited with founding the first school of nursing. The Nightingale School for Nurses was created by Nightingale in England in 1860 and was based on what has been commonly termed as the "Nightingale Principles." The mission of this nursing program was to train nurses who would be prepared to care for patients in their homes and in hospitals (Hunt, 2013; Neeb, 2006). Eventually, schools of nursing were developed in the United States and were modeled on the same principles as Nightingale's school. For example, the Bellevue Training School for Nurses was established in New York City in 1873 (McCloskey & Grace, 1981, as cited in Hunt, 2013). Since that time formalized nursing programs have been developed in every country and although they have changed throughout the years, many of them still follow the basic principles that were developed by Florence Nightingale. Although Florence Nightingale is one of the most widely known and respected founders of modern nursing it is important to note that in the early 1800s there were other training programs for nurses in existence. For example, in 1798, a series of lectures on the care of maternity patients was taught to nurses by Valentine Seaman, who was a physician. Between 1839 and 1850, The Nursing Society of Philadelphia also trained women to provide home care for women during and after childbirth.

There are approximately 3 million nurses in the United States alone and approximately 19.3 million nurses and midwives worldwide (WHO, 2010). Despite these significant numbers, according to the WHO (2010) there remains a worldwide nursing shortage, especially in developing countries. Nursing shortages usually are cyclical in nature and may appear geographically, both internationally and within the United States. Currently, many experts predict a continuing U.S. shortage, including such factors as the Affordable Care Act (ACA), the aging nursing workforce, the faculty shortage, and the ever-increasing older population (American Association of Colleges of Nurses [AACN], 2014). In the United States, there are over 600 baccalaureate programs (Amos, 2005), and approximately 800 associate degree programs (McCaffrey, 2002); however, due to a shortage of faculty and lack of sufficient clinical placements, 79,659 qualified nursing student applicants were denied admission (AACN, 2014).

Today nursing education programs must meet regulatory and accrediting requirements set forth by the licensure and accrediting agencies in their countries. In the United States, programs are regulated by their state boards of education, which use the standards of the National Council of the State Boards of Nursing. The two major accrediting organizations are the Accreditation Commission for Education in Nursing (ACEN), which was formerly known as the National League for Nursing Accreditation Commission (NLNAC), the accrediting body of the National League for Nursing (NLN), and the Commission on Collegiate Nursing Education (CCNE), which is the accrediting body of the AACN. The ACEN may accredit diploma, undergraduate, and graduate programs. The CCNE accredits bachelor of science in nursing (BSN) and graduate nursing programs. As a nursing student you should be sure that you are enrolled in an accredited program. If your program has CCNE accreditation, then you should read the *Essentials of Baccalaureate Education for Professional Nursing Practice*, which is available online. If your program has ACEN accreditation, then you should read their accreditation manual, which can also be located online. Both of these websites contain a wealth of information related to nursing and nursing education.

There are nine main essentials that all CCNE accredited programs must use as a guide when developing their programs and curriculum. These essentials relate to the educational requirements and role of the nurse generalist and focus on leadership, patient outcomes, scholarship and evidenced-based practice, health care policy, interprofessional communication and collaboration, and professionalism. The ACEN (2014; formerly NLNAC) has six major standards that schools must use as a guide when developing their programs and curriculum. These standards relate to the mission of the program, its leadership, faculty, students, resources, and patient outcomes. There are different standards for different programs but they are somewhat similar. Both of these agencies keep abreast of advances in health care and revise their standards as needed. The major difference is that unlike the ACEN, the CCNE does not accredit diploma or associate degree programs. The professional organizations, AACN and NLN, also conduct and fund research, provide educational offerings, and offer certification programs. Most schools of nursing are part of a college or university. In the United States colleges and universities are accredited by one of the following accrediting agencies:

■ Middle State Association of Colleges and Schools (Commission on Higher Education)

- New England Association of Schools and Colleges (Commission on Technical and Career Institutions and Commission on Institutions of Higher Education)
- North Central Association of Colleges and Schools (The Higher Learning Commission, a Commission of the North Central Association)
- Northwest Association of Schools and Colleges
- Southern Association of Colleges and Schools (Commission on Colleges)
- Western Association of Schools and Colleges (Accrediting Commission for Community and Junior Colleges and Accrediting Commission for Senior Colleges and Universities).

Therefore, your college or university will be accredited by one of the agencies listed above and your nursing program will be accredited by CCNE or ACEN. If you are attending a nursing program outside of the United States you should do some research about the regulatory and accrediting agencies that govern your program.

Some of the recent curricula changes in basic nursing programs have been based on advances in health care and technology and current research findings. In recent years there has been a greater emphasis on care of the geriatric/elderly client, including palliative and end-of-life care, quality and safety education for nurses (QSEN) competencies, genetics, the use of evidenced-based practice, and interprofessional collaboration. You want to be sure that the program you attend has updated its curriculum to include the current standards of care and practice.

The ACEN standards and criteria for accrediting baccalaureate nursing programs are similar. For example, Standard 4.4 states "The curriculum includes cultural, ethnic, and socially diverse concepts and may also include experiences from regional, national, or global perspectives" (NLNAC, 2008, p. 4). The curriculum and instructional processes reflect:

- Educational theory
- Interdisciplinary collaboration
- Research and best-practice standards while allowing for innovation and flexibility
- Technological advances

A link to both the ACEN and the CCNE sites is included in the references list for you to read and review in greater detail depending on which one your program received its accreditation from.

Although schools of nursing must meet licensure and accrediting requirements their theoretical framework, philosophical beliefs, and curriculum are unique to each program. Furthermore, the curriculum must be continually reviewed and revised to meet the ever-changing field of nursing and health care. Today, more than ever, schools of nursing use quantitative and qualitative research to evaluate their programs and student outcomes. As a new nursing student you will want to familiarize yourself with your program's curriculum and framework. In fact some students select a school based on the theoretical and philosophical beliefs that guide the curriculum.

ROLE OF NURSE GENERALIST

Nursing is both an art and a science, and is somewhat unique as it is both a practice and a professional discipline. Most basic nursing programs prepare students for the role of nurse generalist. According to Castledine (1996), in Europe most nurses are prepared for the generalist domain, which is the fundamental domain of nursing. During postregistration, nurses often go on to specialize in a particular area. Roles for the baccalaureate generalist nurse are derived from the discipline of nursing. The roles of the baccalaureate generalist include:

- Provider of care
- Designer/manager/coordinator of care
- Member of a profession (American Association of Colleges of Nursing, 2008)

The nurse generalist is expected to provide inpatient and outpatient care to a diverse group of individuals, families, groups, and populations. Nursing practice is informed by a wide variety of disciplines and is based on theory, research, and nursing knowledge. Nursing faculty teach students to understand the discipline of nursing and prepare them for their future roles.

The nurse generalist is prepared to care for culturally diverse patients across the lifespan in a variety of settings, is expected to provide holistic nursing care that is based on evidence, and to promote positive patient outcomes (AACN, 2008).

NURSE PRACTICE ACT AND CODE OF ETHICS

Nursing programs are guided by legal, ethical, and moral codes so it is vital that all nurses understand how these codes impact nursing practice. First and foremost, all nursing students and registered nurses should be well versed in their organization's Nurse Practice Act. In the United States the NCSBN has developed a model Nurse Practice Act and Scope of Practice guidelines for individual state boards of nursing to use as a guide for developing their own Nurse Practice Acts. Because registered nurses are licensed professionals they are legally, morally, and ethically obligated to follow their Nurse Practice Act and Scope of Practice standards.

The NCSBN is a not-for-profit organization whose purpose is to provide an organization through which boards of nursing act and counsel together on matters of common interest and concern affecting public health, safety, and welfare, including the development of licensing examinations in nursing (NCSBN, 2013).

In addition to licensing examinations the NCSBN has developed the Model State Nurse Practice Act definition of nursing (Article 1, Section 1) and each state uses this model as a basis for developing its own unique definition. The Nurse Practice Act provides a broad definition of the roles and responsibilities of all registered professional nurses. According to the NCSBN nurses are required to provide patient-centered care and assist them in achieving optimal health. Visit their website along with your state's website for your state's Nurse Practice Act and additional information about the profession.

Individual countries around the globe also have professional boards of nursing that regulate nursing practice and promote high standards in training, education, and professional conduct. If you reside outside of the United States you should review your country's or province's Nurse Practice Act.

Nursing practice is also informed by the Code of Ethics. For example, in the United States the Code of Ethics can be traced back to 1926 (Viens, 1989). Since that time the Code of Nursing Ethics has undergone several revisions, with the most recent published by the American Nurses Association in 2001 (ANA, 2013). The ANA is in the process of updating its Code of Ethics to reflect current advances in health care and technology.

There is also an International Code of Nursing Ethics that was initially published in 1953; the most current version was released in 2012. The purpose of this code is to guide nurse practice on a global level and is considered a "guide for action based on social values and needs"

International Council of Nurses (ICN, 2012, p. 4). The Code is revised every several years to address current issues in health care from a global perspective. "The Code makes it clear that inherent in nursing is respect for human rights, including the right to life, to dignity and to be treated with respect" (ICN, 2012, p. 1).

The nature of nursing and health care is one that is constantly changing and with each new advance new ethical issues may arise. Therefore it is imperative for all nurses to know these codes and practice in accordance with them. The nursing profession is extremely complex and nurses must also be knowledgeable about the legal, moral, and ethical issues they will face on a daily basis. These issues will be discussed in greater detail in Chapter 6.

LICENSURE REQUIREMENTS

To become a nurse one must successfully pass a licensure exam (see Chapter 7). In the United States the NCSBN sets forth educational and licensure requirements with each state developing its own specific guidelines. In the United States nurses who wish to work in different states are not required to re-take a licensure exam. They only need to apply for reciprocity. However, nurses who wish to work in other countries will have to take the licensure exam offered by that particular country. The NCSBN has developed a Transition Into Practice model to help new nurses transition from "novice to expert" practitioner.

NCSBN TRANSITION INTO PRACTICE MODEL

The NCSBN developed the Transition Into Practice (TIP) model because of the challenges faced by new nurses as they transition into their professional practice roles and in response to issues of patient safety. The model incorporates the use of preceptors and self-learning modules.

The five transition modules include communication and teamwork, patient-centered care, evidenced-based practice, quality improvement, and informatics. Threads that will be integrated throughout the modules include clinical reasoning and safety. These modules incorporate the IOM competencies and specifics for the modules were identified from the literature and from successful transition programs (NCSBN, 2013).

In addition to the transition module there is also one for the preceptors and one for the employers on how to support new nurses.

The TIP has six guiding principles with the overarching goal of promoting public safety by supporting new nurses as they transition into professional practice. According to the NCSBN (2013), transition programs should be developed in collaboration with regulatory agencies, education, and practice and should provide nurses with the knowledge, skills, and attitudes required to deliver safe and effective care.

The program is designed for a period of 6 months but it is the hope of the NSCBN that it will extend for at least a year. They also note that there is flexibility in the program and there will be ongoing evaluations. The TIP model is currently being pilot tested in various hospitals in North Carolina, Ohio, and Illinois. A research study is also being conducted to evaluate the efficacy of this model and its effect on patient safety and outcomes.

IDENTIFY KEY COMPONENTS OF THE INSTITUTE OF MEDICINE *FUTURE OF NURSING* REPORT

There are many organizations that seek to improve health care delivery systems. In the United States the IOM, the Robert Wood Johnson Foundation, and the Jonas Foundation have all played a significant role in this endeavor. Many of their initiatives have had a major influence on the nursing profession. For example, in 2008 the IOM and the Robert Wood Johnson Foundation began a 2-year initiative to respond to the need to assess and transform the nursing profession. The IOM's *The Future of Nursing* report is a must read for all nurses; we are all called on to act both individually and collectively so that we can bring to fruition the goals set forth by our esteemed colleagues. You are entering the profession of nursing during a most exciting time. Because of our past and present influential nurse leaders and educators and the organizations that value and support us we are poised to bring the profession of nursing to new heights. *The Future of Nursing* report was released in 2010; currently individual states are focused on implementing the recommendations set forth in the report.

The four key recommendations are:

- Nurses should use all of their training and education in practice
- Nurses should seek educational improvement and training through educational systems that encourage progression
- Nurses should be considered equal teammates in reconstructing health care in the United States
- Policy making and labor force planning need improved methods for data collection and an information infrastructure (IOM, 2010)

The full report (see reference list) outlines eight recommendations that relate to the four messages. The recommendations include increasing the number of BSN-prepared nurses to 80% by 2020, and doubling the number of doctorally prepared nurses. Expanding scope of practice for nurses is another major goal. Following *The Future of Nursing* report, the Robert Wood Johnson Foundation, in collaboration with the AARP, created the *Future of Nursing Campaign in Action* to promote implementation of the key messages and recommendations. To accomplish this goal they invited several states to be pilots for the action coalitions because each state is governed by different rules and regulations in regard to professional licensure and scope of practice. Currently, all of the states have their own action coalitions, which have a dedicated leadership. In New York there are identified leaders who oversee and collaborate with seven regional action coalitions. The regional action coalitions are comprised of volunteer nurses, nurse educators, nurse leaders, and student nurses. Each action coalition works together to implement the standards set forth in the IOM's *Future of Nursing* report. There is wide support for this endeavor and many organizations are supporting this with funding. For example, the Tri-Council for Nursing, consisting of the American Association of Colleges of Nursing, NLN, American Nurses Association, and the American Organization of Nurse Executives (AONE, 2014) are leading an initiative to create a more educated nursing workforce with funding of $4.3 million from the Robert Wood Johnson Foundation, to assist regional and state coalitions in achieving this goal. They will also offer states that have met or exceeded their benchmarks an additional two years of funding (RWJF, 2012). Clearly, this is a work in progress and it will take both time hard work to implement all the key messages and recommendations. Furthermore, health care is never static so *The Future of Nursing* will always need to be updated and the standards will need to be revised on an ongoing basis. As a student nurse, or newly minted nurse, it is important to get involved to help shape the future of your profession.

CAREER PATHS

There are a multitude of career paths a nurse can follow. "The world is your oyster" when it comes to selecting a career path in nursing. Literally, there is something for everyone. Although many new nurses begin their careers in a hospital setting in direct patient care this is not a requirement. You may work in a hospital or community setting. Of course, depending on your career goals you may have to continue your education and gain more experience before you follow a particular career path. For example, if you aspire to become a nurse manager you will first need to work on a unit and eventually will need to continue your formal education. Although you may not know where you want to specialize it is a good idea to make a 5-year plan outlining at least your initial goals (see Chapter 20).

The following are examples of career paths one might consider if a career in hospital-based nursing is desired (many of these positions require additional experience and education):

- Medical–Surgical
- Pediatrics
- Mother/Baby or Labor and Delivery
- Critical Care
- Operating Room/Postanesthesia Care Unit
- Hemodialysis
- Interventional Cardiology
- Ambulatory Care
- Utilization Review
- Performance Improvement
- Infection Control
- Occupational Health
- Nursing Administration

Some hospitals will require new nurses to work in medical–surgical units but many offer internships or fellowship programs for new nurses who have maintained a high grade point average (GPA) and have strong recommendations, or have completed an externship prior to graduation. Many hospitals prefer to promote from within the organization and will mentor new nurses who are interested in transferring to a specialty unit or aspire to be an administrator or educator.

Examples of nursing roles outside of the hospital include:

- Home care nurses
- Public health nursing
- Flight nursing
- Travel nurses
- Forensic nurses
- Nurse practitioners
- Nurses in the media
- Academic nurse educators
- Nurse authors
- Nurse executives
- Nurse consultants

These are just examples of some of the opportunities that await you. Although these positions require advanced education and several years of experience, with determination and hard work you can obtain one of these positions in the future.

As a nurse you can work almost anywhere in the world. You can work the day shift, evening shift, or night shift. You can work 8-hour shifts, 10-hour shifts, or 12-hour shifts. You can work per diem, part time, or full time. New nurses do not have as many choices as experienced nurses but after a couple of years you can become more selective. With the *Future of Nursing* initiatives, the Affordable Care Act, and advancing science and technology, the role of the nurse will continue to expand and new opportunities will arise with each passing year.

SUMMARY

This introductory chapter included an overview of professional nursing practice. An overview of the regulatory and accrediting agencies that inform nursing practice was presented. The significance of the Nurse Practice Act and Code of Ethics was also discussed in addition to the role of the NCSBN. *The Future of Nursing* report and Campaign for Action were also discussed and a list of potential career paths was presented.

DISCUSSION QUESTIONS

1. Explain the role of the nurse generalist.
2. What are the key components of the Nurse Practice Act?
3. What is the difference between the ANA's Code of Ethics and the International Code of Ethics?
4. Describe the NCSBN's Transition Into Practice Model.
5. What are the four key messages in *The Future of Nursing* report?
6. List and discuss three future nursing roles.
7. What are the eight recommendations of the IOM's *The Future of Nursing* report?
8. What are the educational paths you can take to become a registered nurse?
9. Discuss the significant contributions of Florence Nightingale.
10. What is Mary Seacole known for in nursing?

Suggested Learning Activities

* Locate copies of the Nurse Practice Act, Code of Ethics, and the NCLEX-RN® plan.
* Write a two-page essay comparing and contrasting the ANA's *Code of Ethics* and the International Code of Ethics.
* Compare the model Nurse Practice Act with your state's Nurse Practice Act. Give a 3-to 5-minute presentation to your classmates.

REFERENCES

American Association of Colleges of Nursing. (2008). *The essentials of baccalaureate education for professional nursing practice.* Retrieved from http://www.AACN.com

American Association of Colleges of Nursing. (2014). *Nursing shortage.* Retrieved from http://www.aacn.nche.edu

American Nurses Association. (2001). *Code of ethics for nurses.* Retrieved from http://www.nursingworld.org/codeofethics

Amos, L. (2005). *American Association of Colleges of Nursing. Baccalaureate nursing programs.* Retrieved from http://www.AACN.com

Castledine, G. (1996). Castledine column. The value of the generalist nursing domain. *British Journal of Nursing, 5*(18), 1146.

Fairman, J. (2012). History for the future (of nursing). *Nursing History Review, 20*(1), 10–13. doi:10.1891/1062-8061.20.10

Hunt, D. (2013). *The new nurse educator: Mastering academe.* New York: Springer Publishing.

Institute of Medicine. (2010). *The future of nursing: Leading change, advancing health.* Retrieved from http://www.iom.edu

International Council of Nurses. (2012). *ICN code of ethics for nurses.* Retrieved from http://www.icn.ch/about-icn/code-of-ethics-for-nurses/

Jarrín, O. (2010). Core elements of U.S. Nurse Practice Acts and incorporation of nursing diagnosis language. *International Journal of Nursing Terminologies & Classifications, 21*(4), 166–176. doi:10.1111/j.1744-618X.2010.01162.x

McCaffey, E. (2002). The relevance of associate degree nursing education: Past, present, future. *Online Journal of Issues in Nursing, 7* (2), Manuscript 2. Retrieved from http://www.nursingworld.org/ojin/MainMenuCategories/ANAMarketplace/ANAPeriodicals/OJIN/TableofContents/Volume72002/No2May2002/RelevanceofAssociateDegree.aspx

McCloskey, J., & Grace, H. (1981). *Current issues in nursing.* Oxford, UK: Blackwell

National Council of State Boards of Nursing. (2013). *Nursing regulation in the U.S.* Retrieved from https://www.ncsbn.org/

National League for Nurses Accreditation Commission. (2008). *Scientific publications. NLNAC 2008 standards and criteria – Baccalaureate.* Retrieved from http://www.acenursing.net/manuals/sc2008_baccalaureate.pdf

Neeb, K. (2006). *Mental health nursing.* (3rd ed). Philadelphia, PA: F.A. Davis Company.

Robert Wood Johnson Foundation. (2012). *Robert Wood Johnson Foundation launches initiative to support academic progression in nursing.* Retrieved at http://www.rwjf.org

Toman, C., & Thifault, M. C. (2012). Historical thinking and the shaping of nursing identity. *Nursing History Review, 20,* 184–204. doi:http://dx.doi.org.ezproxy.cnr.edu/10.1891/1062-8061.20.184

Viens, D. C. (1989). A history of nursing's code of ethics. *Nursing Outlook, 37* (1), 45–49. Retrieved from www.sandiego.edu

World Health Organization. (2010). Wanted: 2.4 million nurses, and that's just in India. *Bulletin Of the World Health Organization, 88*(5), 321–400.

World Health Organization. (2011). *World health statistics.* Retrieved from http://www.who.com

CHAPTER 2

Academic Foundations for Your Future Role

Our greatest glory is not in never failing, but in rising up every time we fail.

—Ralph Waldo Emerson

OBJECTIVES

After reading this chapter, the reader will be able to:

- Discuss the relationship of academic success to one's future professional role
- Identify strategies for academic success
- Understand the importance of learning styles
- Understand the significance of academic integrity
- Understand the significance of grade point average (GPA) and its future role
- Use social media and Internet etiquette
- Understand the significance of externships and internships on future role attainment

The foundation and/or building blocks of any profession are vital to one's success. This is especially true in nursing because of the complexity of the role of the nurse and health care in general. Your foundation began long before you entered nursing school. In fact it began the day you were born. All of your past life experiences will help to shape your future role as a nurse. For example, as a nursing student you will need good study habits so that you can achieve academic success. Some of you may have already mastered this, but others will need to develop better study habits. Nursing school is very challenging and requires hours of hard work and preparation. This chapter will review many strategies for success. In addition to academic success and academic integrity there are other areas, such as networking, social media, externships, and internships, that will have a positive impact on your transition into professional practice.

RELATIONSHIP OF ACADEMIC SUCCESS
TO YOUR PROFESSIONAL ROLE

The journey you take as a student will have a major impact on your future role as a nurse. This journey will require many hours of didactic classes and clinical experiences. You will spend hours reading, studying, researching, practicing clinical skills, and writing. Each semester your course work will become more challenging. Therefore, developing strategies for academic success as soon as possible is extremely important. Harsh as it may sound there is little room for failure in nursing school. Although each school has different policies, some schools do not allow for any failures in a nursing/theory course. Furthermore, today's job market is highly competitive and employers are very selective when hiring new nurses. Many hospitals set a minimum GPA (3.0–3.5) to be considered for an externship, internship, fellowship, or a staff nurse position. Therefore, it is vital for you to employ all the strategies available to foster your success. Externships are very valuable and are available to nursing students who meet the criteria. The selection process is very competitive and you will not even be considered if your GPA is below the requirement. Externships provide students with a 6- to 8-week clinical experience during the summer and you are paired up with a preceptor and also attend didactic classes every week. After the formal externship many students are hired as per diem nursing assistants until they graduate. Completing an externship provides you with invaluable experience and is also looked on favorably by nurse recruiters.

An internship, residency, or fellowship is offered to new graduate nurses who have excelled in their nursing program, although many require that you obtain your license prior to hire. The length of these preceptored programs varies from 6 months to 1 year in a specialty area and is extremely beneficial as you transition to professional practice.

There are many factors that relate to academic success in a nursing program. Higgins (2005) found that students who have strong grades in reading, writing, and math, and maintain a GPA above 2.5 in biology, anatomy, and physiology, were more likely to successfully complete their nursing programs. There is also a relationship between course grades, and passing the National Council Licensure Examination (NCLEX-RN®). For example, McGahee et al. (2010) posits that course grades, especially in science and foundational courses, are positively related to NCLEX success in baccalaureate students—thus emphasizing the importance of developing strategies that will foster academic success.

IDENTIFY STRATEGIES FOR ACADEMIC SUCCESS

There are many strategies that nursing students may undertake in order to be successful both academically and clinically. Many of these strategies will pertain to both areas, whereas others will relate specifically to the academic or clinical setting. A major strategy is to do the best that you can do in all of your courses because they all are geared to your holistic development. Of course, this is easier said than done, and some courses will require more effort than others, however, it is important to develop a plan that will enable you to manage your course load. Furthermore, if you do not believe that you can be successful with a full course load then you should consider attending on a part-time basis. Most programs provide students with an academic advisor who can guide them in the right direction. The nursing program is very demanding and there are strict policies regarding progression and passing/ failing a course. For example, some programs allow only one failure in a theory/clinical course. Additionally, passing requirements are often more stringent than normal, with a C+ or B being the minimum grade for passing the course. Even though the minimum grade may be a C+ you should strive to earn the best grade possible, not only for your GPA but for your long-term knowledge development and synthesis. You need to figure out how all of the theoretical knowledge you are acquiring relates to the care of your patients, who will be similar yet different to the textbook cases you learn about. This requires a thorough understanding of all the science and nursing courses you will complete before you graduate.

The following strategies may be helpful in fostering success in your academic journey:

- Thoroughly reviewing the course syllabus and outlines
- Developing a weekly outline with goals, objectives, and requirements for each course

■ Developing a weekly checklist
■ Completing all reading and written assignments in a timely fashion
■ Meeting with course faculty to discuss progress and strategies
■ Participating in simulations
■ Spending time in the skills lab
■ Joining a study group
■ Using all available resources (faculty advisor, the library, tutoring, writing center, etc.)
■ Practicing NCLEX questions
■ Knowing your preferred learning style
■ Keeping a journal
■ Participating in self-care activities
■ Joining a support group
■ Developing time management and organizational skills
■ Seeking out a mentor
■ Considering part-time course work if full time is too overwhelming

When you begin each semester you should develop a plan for success. This will require time, dedication, motivation, persistence, perseverance, time-management skills, and organization. First you need to read each course syllabus carefully and be sure to understand the expectations and outcomes. Clarification with your teacher is vital. You should purchase the textbooks as soon as possible. Next you should develop a weekly schedule for each of your classes and include all the required assignments. Then you should figure out how much time you will need to complete each assignment—reading, writing, and studying. Once you develop the plan you should try to follow it as closely as possible. You can devise a daily, weekly, monthly, or semester plan; however, weekly is recommended so as not to feel overwhelmed. You may also want to develop a checklist and check off each item as you complete it. This is a great motivator and helps you to stay on task.

This is certainly not an all-inclusive list, however, following these tips and strategies will help you to have a successful academic journey. It is important to note that learning is an individual experience and therefore some strategies will work better than others. You will also want to continue to use tried-and-true strategies that you have found helpful in your previous educational experiences. Nursing school is very challenging and you need to start off on the right foot so you don't miss out on the important building blocks that may be found throughout your program.

ACADEMIC INTEGRITY

There are many issues that relate to academic integrity and it is important not to engage in any practice that may be viewed as academic dishonesty. Academic integrity is the act of completing one's own work whether it is homework, an exam, or a scholarly paper. "Academic integrity is defined as 'a commitment, even in the face of adversity, to five fundamental values: honesty, trust, fairness, respect, and responsibility" (Cleary et al., 2013, p. 264). Breaches of academic integrity have become more prevalent in recent years and include all forms of cheating and plagiarism. Woith et al. (2013) posits that academic dishonesty is increasing in all students, including nursing students despite the factor that the nursing profession has been identified as one of the most trusted professions for the past several years. Furthermore, students who breach academic integrity are more likely to engage in illegal or unethical behavior. Park et al. (2013) found similar issues in nursing students from South Korea. Woith et al. (2013) described several factors that are related to academic dishonesty among student nurses which relate to students, faculty, and systems. Student factors include engaging in unethical behavior and using technology to engage in academic dishonesty, in addition to placing patients at risk due to covering up errors, falsifying patient records, and failing to question incorrect orders. Faculty issues relate to unrealistic content and failure to address breaches, although many faculty do incorporate a variety of strategies and consequences to prevent academic dishonesty. System issues relate to large class sizes, inadequate socialization into the profession, and accelerated programs. Most students do value and understand the importance of academic integrity and faculty must continue to implement measures to deter academic dishonesty, which should also be addressed in tandem with lectures on incivility (Woith et al. 2013). Sometimes students do not realize they have engaged in academic dishonesty due to a lack of knowledge. For example, a student who is accused of plagiarism may not have intended to do so, but did not know how to cite properly. Always consult with the writing center or your faculty for guidance on writing scholarly papers with proper citations and references. Culture may play a role as students may have been taught to help each other, so they may not realize that sharing a paper with another student could be viewed as a breach of academic integrity. According to Tippitt et al. (2009) "Unethical behaviors in the classroom and clinical settings by nursing students includes the following: lying, cheating, sharing information via any means possible, plagiarizing the work of others, falsifying information on patients' charts, and fabricating home visits" (p. 240). These are very serious issues and you certainly do not want to knowingly engage in any of these practices, which are highly unethical and may result in failure or dismissal from your nursing program. Furthermore, falsifying patient medical records or fabricating home visits is illegal. Nursing school is very challenging and you may feel pressured to engage in academic dishonesty by other students, however, you must always be guided by your conscience and never engage in deleterious behaviors, especially ones that place your patient at risk. Ignorance is not an excuse, so be sure to understand the behaviors and actions that would constitute a breach of academic integrity. Furthermore, if someone is trying to coerce you into engaging in an activity that is unethical you should consult with either your teacher, faculty advisor, or an administrator.

LEARNING STYLES

Learning styles relate to an individual's preferred method of learning. They include the domains of auditory, visual, and kinesthetic learning and although most individuals use all three of three of these domains of learning there is often a dominant or preferred domain. "Learning is a unique experience for every person. Many factors contribute to how a person learns and although learning takes place in a multifaceted way most learners have a preferred learning style" (Hunt, 2013, chapter 7, p. 1). There are many theories and a plethora of literature that describe and explain how one learns. "Learners' visual, auditory, and kinesthetic learning preferences are the central focus of the perceptions approach to determining learning styles" (Merriam, Caffarella, & Baumgartner, 2007, p. 408). Learning styles include visual, auditory, kinesthetic, logical, social, solitary, and experiential (Brady, 2013). Some learners are visual learners, whereas others are auditory. Some learners are more "hands on" and need to do something physical to actually learn it. For example, you might watch a video and a demonstration on inserting a Foley catheter, but need to actually perform the skill before you learn it. You will also benefit greatly from simulation experiences. Mastery of content requires reinforcement, review, and practice thus most individuals need a variety of styles to learn. However, it is very helpful to know what your preferred style of learning is so that you can optimize your learning. For example, if you are an auditory learner you may want to bring a tape recorder to class so you can record your instructor and listen to the recordings as many times as you need. Of course, you need to check with your faculty member because some faculty are not comfortable with having their lectures taped. Some faculty may provide you with a taped version of the lecture or post it on their course management system. If your faculty does not wish to be recorded you can always make your own recording from your notes and textbook. Some electronic textbooks also have an audio option. Visual learners need to read and review chapters, notes, PowerPoint presentations, and other visual aids. Logical learners need to reason out information to learn it. Social learners prefer group learning, thus a study group is very helpful to them, whereas solitary learners prefer to learn and study by themselves. Kolb (1984, 1999), described four types of learning styles/preferences in his experiential model—diverging, assimilating, converging, and accommodating—and developed the Learning Styles Inventory (LSI) to measure these different styles. The diverging learner is both concrete and reflective and prefers to learn in groups. An assimilating learner is an abstract and reflective learner who likes to build models and test theories. The converging learner is abstract and active and prefers practical applications and problem solving. An accommodating learner is concrete and active and likes to engage in trial and error and intuitively solves problems. Completing a learning styles assessment can help you to determine your preferred method of learning. You can complete an online learning styles assessment at https://www.learningstyles.com ("Overview of Learning Styles," 2011). Most faculty use a variety of teaching and learning strategies that include the three domains of learning; however, you need to supplement and develop strategies based on your individual needs and preferred methods of learning.

Some researchers have examined the relationship between learning styles and critical thinking in addition to the preferred learning styles of undergraduate nurses. For example, Andreou et al. (2014) completed a review of the literature to examine the relationship between learning styles and critical-thinking skills and found that there may be a relationship; however, this warrants further investigation. Critical thinking is another important skill for students and nurses to develop, thus this is an important study in regards to development of critical-thinking and reasoning skills. In an earlier study, An and Yoo (2008) examined the learning styles of undergraduate nursing students using the LSI, which describes four types of learning modes—concrete experience (CE), reflective observation (RO), abstract conceptualization (AC), and active experimentation (AE). There are four learning styles related to the learning modes: accommodating, diverging, assimilating, and converging. An and Yu concluded, "The learning styles of undergraduate nursing students in Korea were mainly diverging and accommodating" (p. 107). This study may apply to the undergraduate nursing population in general, or only to the sample, or only to students with similar characteristics to the sample in this study. Clearly learning style is related to student outcomes so it is important to identify your dominant style of learning.

An important role of all nurses is that of patient educator and one must also understand the learning styles of one's patients. Tailoring your education to a patient's preferred learning style can improve the patient education experience (Brady, 2013). Patient education requires sharing knowledge that is easy to understand and based on the health literacy and learning styles. "Because education and literacy levels vary among patients most experts agree that teaching materials should be geared to a 6th to 8th grade reading level and jargon should be avoided" (Canobbio, 2006, as cited in Hunt, 2013, p. 26). Many organizations have well-developed patient education materials that you can use when teaching your patients, and you will certainly have opportunities as a student and during your orientation to learn more about patient education and to try various methods. However, learning styles of patients are not usually considered when engaging in patient education.

LEARNING NEEDS AND ACCOMMODATIONS

Many students have special learning needs and require certain accommodations to help them to be successful in school. Nursing students are among those and although you may be hesitant to self-identify it is the only way you will be given accommodations. There are many legal issues that relate to disabilities and if you have a disability you must be knowledgeable about the accommodations you can expect as a student and a nurse. The important thing is to self-identify if you feel you need accommodations. If you receive accommodations in high school than you will most likely need them in college. However, there is a process you must follow with your school that requires formal testing by a licensed practitioner. In accordance with the Americans with Disabilities Act, organizations are required to make reasonable accommodations (Carroll, 2004).

> The Americans with Disabilities Act (ADA) was developed to protect the rights of people with disabilities. It was originally created in 1973 as the Rehabilitation Act and went through several revisions and endorsements. In 1990 the Rehabilitation Act of 1973 was amended to reflect the principles of the ADA which resulted in the Americans with Disabilities Act and Section 504 being signed into law in July of 1990. The most recent endorsement of the Americans with Disabilities Act Amendments Act of 2008 was signed by President Bush with additional revisions signed by the Attorney General in 2010. (ADA, 2011, as cited in Hunt, 2013, p. 251)

Students have the right to privacy and only their faculty members know of their special needs, which may be related to a learning disability or a physical disability. Individualized accommodations are developed based on a formal assessment and recommendations from the licensed provider in consultation with student services and the student. Maheady (2003) posits, "Faculty members should consider the development of an Individual Nursing Education Program for every nursing student with a disability, similar to those used with special education students in public schools" (p. 154). Accommodations may include extended testing time, testing in a different location, use of technology, specialized equipment such as amplified stethoscopes, scribes, recorded lectures, modified clinical assignments, Braille notes, and preferred seating (Arndt, 2004, as cited in Hunt, 2013). Nurses with special needs can work in a variety of settings such as home care, case management, parish nurse, nursing research, and a host of other areas (Evans, 2005; Maheady, 1999). Being your own advocate is extremely important because unfortunately some nurses and faculty may unknowingly or knowingly discriminate against students with disabilities, which is often related to lack of knowledge and/or well-developed policies. Only you can decide whether or not you want to self-identify and receive the benefits related to accommodations in addition to the laws that protect you. It will also be important to apply for accommodations when taking the NCLEX as you want to do everything in your power to be successful. Remember you are legally protected from discrimination under the Americans with Disabilities Act, and you need to self-identify as soon as possible to receive accommodations. If you wait until you are failing or fail a course it will be too late to change the outcome. The decision on whether or not to apply for accommodations is yours to make; however, do not make the decision until you have carefully weighed the positive and negative issues associated with your decision. It is helpful to consult with your family and mentors. Each academic organization has its own specific policies and procedures so be sure to review these carefully. Your faculty member can only provide you with the accommodations that have been officially approved by your college or university.

PROFESSIONAL BEHAVIOR

Professional behavior as a student and later as a nurse is extremely important and required of all individuals who belong to a profession. The way you conduct yourself reflects on you as an individual, your school, and the nursing profession.

Professionalism is expected and required of all practice disciplines. For example, "Professionalism in Physical Therapy: Core Values features seven elements: accountability, altruism, compassion/caring, excellence, integrity, professional duty, and social responsibility" (Ries, 2013, p. 19). These core values are certainly applicable to nurses, too. Being accountable for one's actions is very important in nursing. For example, you need to be prepared and competent and if you make an error you need to report it and ensure that the patient is provided with the appropriate treatment. Altruism relates to being selfless and helping others—nursing is a giving profession and requires much dedication. Compassion and caring are at the core of nursing and you need to treat all patients and families with the utmost respect. Excellence relates to your knowledge, competence, and critical thinking and reasoning. Patients have a right to expect a professional and competent nurse. Integrity is foundational to your behavior as a student and a nurse and precludes you from engaging in deleterious behavior. Professional duty relates to being present and punctual, adhering to your job description, completing your assignments, and collaborating with the interprofessional team. Social responsibility relates to engaging in activities of social justice and being sure not to engage in social activities that are unlawful or may harm self or others.

Communication in written, verbal, and nonverbal form is related to professional behavior. You want to be sure you use proper grammar, tone, and avoid slang when speaking. Your written documents should always be polished with formal sentences that are grammatically correct. You also want to make sure your nonverbal communication is respectful. Your personal attire and grooming should be neat and clean with minimal make-up and jewelry. Interpersonal relationships are also important and you need to stay calm and professional even when others are acting out. This is not to say that you should allow someone to verbally or physically abuse you, you just need to follow the proper protocols. Although it may be difficult, don't yell or use slang words—instead stay calm and report the situation to your supervisor. Writing about the situation in your journal can help you to cope with your feelings. You also shouldn't discuss your personal problems in the workplace. Your personal image is part of your professional image and it is important to portray yourself in a positive manner. Larson (2006) posits that one of the keys to a successful nursing career is having a positive and professional image. Professionalism has a positive effect on a profession and professionals. For example, Çelik and Hisar (2012) found a positive relationship between professionalism and job satisfaction in nurses. The benefits of professionalism are well documented and you want to be sure to always have a professional image, demeanor, and conduct, which will lead to personal satisfaction, job satisfaction, respect, and role development.

SOCIAL MEDIA

Social media refers to a myriad of online software programs and has positive and negative associations, especially in nursing (Lachman, 2013). There are many wonderful uses for social media, however, you must be careful about the messages and images you share on sites such as Facebook and Twitter. Furthermore, you must always be careful not to discuss your patients, family members, or place of employment online. You must also understand the relationship of the Health Insurance Portability and Accountability Act (HIPAA), confidentiality, social media, and protection of patients' rights (Lachman, 2013). Because of the pervasiveness of this issue the National Council of State Boards of Nursing (NCSBN) published *White Paper: A Nurse's Guide to Social Media* in 2011. This document contains guidelines for all nurses on the use of social media. Although most organizations have very specific social medial policies, typically these pertain to use within the specific organization and do not pertain to personal use. Many nurses have been reported to their State Boards of Nursing due to breaches in their personal use of social media. Confidentiality and protection of privacy are expected of all health care workers, and because nurses have access to the entire medical record and personal information they must be careful not to divulge any information that could potentially identify a patient. Therefore it is important to not engage in posting photos, comments, or complaints about patients, families, coworkers, or your organization. Furthermore, posting negative or harassing comments can be considered a form of online or cyber bullying. According to the National Council of State Boards of Nursing (NCSBN, 2011), nurses may be reported to their Board of Nursing for the following reasons:

- Unprofessional conduct
- Unethical conduct
- Moral turpitude
- Mismanagement of patient records
- Revealing a privileged communication
- Breach of confidentiality

These breaches may lead to disciplinary action such as a reprimand or monetary fine, suspension, or loss of licensure. Even if one is not reported to the Board of Nursing, if an employer discovers that an employee has breached privacy and confidentiality or has spoken negatively about his or her coworkers and/or the hospital, the employer may suspend or terminate the employee. The majority of nurses and other employees who are reprimanded for breaches of confidentiality and privacy do not realize that they have done something wrong. They may feel what they write in their e-mails or on their social media accounts is private. However, this is not the case and especially when using workplace computers as employers have access to all accounts. Therefore, your best policy is to not post anything that could potentially be viewed in a negative way. "Nurses should be mindful of employer policies, relevant state and federal laws, and professional standards regarding patient privacy and confidentiality and its application to social and electronic media" (NCSBN, 2011, p. 3). The American Nurses Association (2011) developed six principles for nurses to follow when engaging in social networking. The principles relate to protection of patient privacy, maintaining boundaries between patients and nurses, and requires nurses to report any violations of patient privacy in regard to the use of social media.

These principles are very clear and all students and nurses should follow them in addition to reading the material published by the National Council of State Boards of Nursing.

This issue is also being addressed around the world with guidelines being developed regarding social media and its use in society. The United Kingdom and Australia have created clear guidelines in response to issues with social media, and New Zealand is collaborating with its education partner to develop similar guidelines (Flutey, 2011). Hospitals and other organizations use social media to share information about their organization, provide patient information, and recruit new members and/or employees. Because social media is still expanding it is difficult to foresee all the potential issues that may result from its use and some organizations do not yet have clear policies in place regarding personal use of social media. Hospitals should develop policies and procedures prior to implementing a web-based program ("Social Media: What Your Hospital Should Know," 2014). It is very important for you to know your organization's policies and procedures, in addition to your state's board of nursing regulations, and the legal, ethical, and moral implications related to the use of social media.

FEATURE: TOP 10 TIPS FOR STUDENTS

1. Enroll in an accredited academic program

2. Develop a close relationship with your faculty advisor

3. Join a study group, be proactive, and stay focused

4. Use all available resources

5. Read and reread your textbooks and articles; take good notes

6. Practice your skills in the learning center

7. Engage in extracurricular activity and self-care activities

8. Find a mentor

9. Engage in activities that focus on critical thinking and reasoning

10. Join a professional organization such as the Student Nurses Association

SUMMARY

This chapter focused on academic success and its relationship to successful completion of nursing school in addition to future opportunities for externships, internships, residencies, and fellowships. Strategies for academic success in addition to the importance of learning styles were also included. The relationship between learning needs and accommodations was briefly discussed. The importance of professionalism in relation to role development was reviewed in addition to potential issues, both positive and negative, related to the use of social media.

DISCUSSION QUESTIONS

1. What is the relationship between academic success and your future nursing role?

2. List and discuss four strategies for academic success.

3. What is the benefit of an externship?

4. What law protects individuals with disabilities?

5. List five accommodations a student with special needs may require.

6. What are the various learning styles?

7. Why is it important to know your learning style?

8. What is professionalism?

9. What are some issues related to the use of social media?

10. What is HIPAA and why is it important?

Suggested Learning Activities

▪ Identify potential organizations for externships/internships and attend one National Student Nurses' Association meeting.
▪ Read your organization's policy on the use of social media.
▪ Interview a nurse about professionalism.
▪ Complete a self-assessment of your learning style.
▪ Develop a plan for your academic success.

REFERENCES

Amdt, M. (2004). Educating nursing students with disabilities: One nurse educator's journey questions to clarity. *Journal of Nursing Education, 43*(5), 204–206.

American Nurses Association (ANA). (2011). *ANA's principles for social networking and the nurse.* Silver Spring, MD: Author. Retrieved from http://www.nursingworld.org/FunctionalMenuCategories/AboutANA/Social-Media/Social-Networking-Principles-Toolkit/6-Tips-for-Nurses-Using-Social-Media-Poster.pdf

An, G., & Yoo, M. (2008). Critical thinking and learning styles of nursing students at the baccalaureate nursing program in Korea. *Contemporary Nurse: A Journal for the Australian Nursing Profession, 29*(1), 100–109.

Andreou, C., Papastavrou, E., & Merkouris, A. (2014). Learning styles and critical thinking relationship in baccalaureate nursing education: A systematic review. *Nurse Education Today, 34*(3), 362–371. doi:10.1016/j.nedt.2013.06.004

Brady, C.L. (2013). Understanding learning styles: Providing the optimal learning experience. *International Journal of Childbirth Education, 28*(2), 16–19.

Canobbio, M.M. (2006). *Mosby's Handbook of patient teaching* (3rd ed.). St. Louis, MO: Mosby.

Carroll, S. (2004). Inclusion of people with physical disabilities in nursing education. *Journal of Nursing Education, 43*(5), 207–212.

Çelik, S., & Hisar, F. (2012). The influence of the professionalism behaviour of nurses working in health institutions on job satisfaction. *International Journal of Nursing Practice, 18*(2), 180–187. doi:10.1111/j.1440-172X.2012.02019.x

Cleary, M., Walter, G., Horsfall, J., & Jackson, D. (2013). Promoting integrity in the workplace: A priority for all academic health professionals.

Contemporary Nurse: A Journal for the Australian Nursing Profession, 45(2), 264–268. doi:10.5172/conu.2013.45.2.264

Evans, B. C. (2005). Nursing education for students with disabilities: Our students, our teachers. In M. Oermann & K. Heinrich (Eds.), *Annual Review of Nursing Education,* (pp. 3–22). New York, NY: Springer Publishing.

Flutey, M. (2011). Using social media cautiously. *Kai Tiaki Nursing New Zealand, 17*(7), 45.

Higgins, B. (2005). Strategies for lowering attrition rates and raising NCLEX-RN pass rates. *Journal of Nursing Education, 44*(12), 541–547.

Hunt, D. (2013). *The New nurse educator: Mastering academe.* New York, NY: Springer Publishing.

Kolb, D. (1984). *Experiential learning: Experience as the source of learning and development.* Englewood Cliffs, N J: Prentice Hall.

Kolb, D. (1999). *The Kolb learning style inventory: Version 3.* Boston, MA: Hay Group.

Lachman, V. D. (2013). Social media: Managing the ethical issues. *Med-Surg Matters, 22*(5), 326–329.

Larson, S. (2006). *Create a good impression: Professionalism in nursing.* Retrieved from http://www.nsna.org/portals/0/skins/nsna/.../imprint_novdec06_feat_larson.pdf

Overview of learning styles. (2011). Retrieved from http://www.learning-styles-online.com/overview

McGahee, T. W., Gramling, L., & Reid, T. F. (2010). NCLEX-RN® success: Are there predictors. *Southern Online Journal of Nursing Research, 10*(4), 208–221.

Maheady, D. (1999). Jumping through hoops, walking on egg shells: The experiences of nursing students with disabilities. *Journal of Nursing Education, 38*(4), 162–170.

Merriam, S. B., Caffarella, R. S., & Baumgartner, L. M. (2007). Memory, cognition, and the brain. In *Learning in adulthood: A comprehensive guide.* (3rd ed.). Hoboken, NJ: Wiley. Retrieved from https://login.ezproxy.cnr.edu/login?qurl=http://www.credoreference.com/entry/wileyla/memory_cognition_and_the_brain.

National Council of State Boards of Nursing. (2011). *White paper: A nurses guide to the use of social media.* Retrieved from http://www.ncsbn.com

Park, E., Park, S., & Jang, I. (2013). Academic cheating among nursing students. *Nurse Education Today, 33*(4), 346–352. doi:10.1016/j.nedt.2012.12.015

Ries, E. (2013). The power of professionalism. *PT in Motion, 5*(8), 16–24.

Social Media: What your hospital should know. (2014). *H&HN: Hospitals & Health Networks, 88*(2), 41–47.

Tippitt, M., Ard, N., Kline, J., Tilghman, J., Chamberlain, B., & Meagher, P. (2009). Creating environments that foster academic integrity. *Nursing Education Perspectives, 30*(4), 239–244.

U. S. Department of Justice. (n.d.). *ADA home page—information and technical assistance.* Retrieved from http://www.ada.gov.

Woith, W., Jenkins, S., & Kerber, C. (2012). Perceptions of academic integrity among nursing students. *Nursing Forum, 47*(4), 253–259. doi:10.1111/j.1744-6198.2012.00274.x

CHAPTER 3

Self-Care, Advocacy, and Resiliency

When we learn how to become resilient, we learn how to embrace the beautifully broad spectrum of the human experience.

—Jaeda DeWalt

OBJECTIVES

After reading this chapter, the reader will be able to:

- Understand the importance of self-care
- Identify self-care strategies
- Understand the relationship between resiliency and success
- Discuss ways to strengthen resiliency
- Understand the relationship of self-advocacy and success.

Nursing is an extremely gratifying profession and as a nurse you will receive many rewards: both intrinsic and extrinsic. However, the journey you will embark on as a student, and eventually as a registered nurse, will be very demanding and at times overwhelming. Throughout your journey you will experience joy and sorrow, confidence and self-doubt, satisfaction and dissatisfaction, and, at times, emotional and physical exhaustion. The impact and significance of these positive and negative experiences will be balanced so that you will be able to persevere. However, there will be times when the negatives may outweigh the positives and vice versa. There is a saying in nursing that in order to take care of others one must first take care of oneself (Trossman, 2013). This chapter will focus on the importance of coping strategies, such as self-care, advocacy, and resiliency in relation to success in your nursing program, and throughout your entire career in nursing. Developing and incorporating these strategies will serve you well as you complete your journey from student to licensed professional nurse. "Stressful working conditions in nursing are a major cause of burnout among nurses. Burnout is characterized by exhaustion, cynicism, and low professional efficacy" (Laschinger & Wong, 2006, p. 358). Becoming more resilient will help you in your personal and professional life. Learning how to engage in self-care and selecting self-care strategies is an important step in being able to care for patients, families, and colleagues. Advocacy is one of the most important roles of the nurse and being able to self-advocate whether in the classroom or clinical setting is vital for your well-being.

SELF-CARE FROM STUDENT TO PROFESSIONAL

Nursing has been described as both an art and a science, with the phenomena of concern being the health and well-being of individuals, families, and groups. Caring is one of the basic tenets of nursing, and holistic nursing care is a major focus in both service (health care organizations) and academia. In fact, many nursing programs include holistic health and caring in the theoretical framework that guides their curriculum. "Caring in nursing is characterized by a holistic view of mankind, and nursing care is directed toward not only providing care for the patient's fundamental needs but also caring for the patient's values and experiences" (Watson, 2008, as cited in Ranheim et al., 2012, p. 79). There is a wealth of information about caring and caring theory in the literature and it is essential to become well acquainted with this subject. Although caring has been described as the "essence of nursing" (Watson, 1988, 2008), self-care has not been given the same attention. Indeed, much of the literature on self-care is based on the patient. For example, Orem's Theory of Self-Care is focused on the patient taking control of his or her health and care outcomes (Orem, 1995). Interestingly, over 25 years ago, McCarthy (1986) identified self-care as an important issue for student nurses in her study on self-care agency. However, this issue has received little attention in the current literature. Nevertheless, one must learn how to care for themselves before he or she can care for others. Furthermore, nursing school is demanding and stressful and students must learn how to cope and engage in self-care (Chow & Kalischuck, 2008). According to Trossman (2013), "Nursing students repeatedly put aside their own health and wellness to get through the rigors of challenging courses and clinical rotations" (p. 1). Many students are under the erroneous assumption that they do not have time to care for themselves. According to Christiaens, a member of the Utah Nurses Association and a well-known speaker, self-care is vitally important when providing holistic nursing care (Trossman, 2013, p. 2).

The American Nurses Association (ANA) and the National Student Nurses' Association are addressing the issue of stress and self-care by developing several key initiatives. For example, the ANA launched the "HealthyNurse" initiative (https://www.nursingworld.org/healthynurse), in 2012. This initiative focuses on the health and well-being of nurses. To that end nurses have online resources available and a multitude of information about health and wellness (Trossman, 2013). Many nurses do not take the time to care for themselves and are not aware of the valuable resources that are available to them. Hence it is important to understand and develop self-care strategies as a student so that they become ingrained in daily practice. "Self-care is an important proactive strategy for nursing students as it may have tremendous influence on student burnout and attrition" (Chow & Kalischuck, 2008, p. 32). According to Kravitz et al. (2010), self-care may also be a factor in reducing stress and burnout in nurses, which has been identified as a significant factor in the nursing shortage. Burnout is often described as something that occurs when an individual does not have the required coping skills when faced with chronic stressors, such as in the nursing profession. When faced with these stressors nurses may employ positive or negative coping strategies. Negative coping strategies include overeating, substance abuse, and smoking, whereas positive strategies include meditation, exercise, and healthy eating. Furthermore, burnout is also associated with high nurse turnover rates (Raingruber & Robinson, 2007), patient dissatisfaction, and decreased quality of care. Therefore, it is extremely important to employ strategies that will decrease burnout and improve patient outcomes. Kravitz et al. (2010) investigated the relationship of psychoeducational interventions in the promotion of self-care strategies in a sample of 189 females and 76 males who were new graduate nurses working in oncology. They found that using formal classroom education and art therapy was positively related with the development of self-care strategies. Based on their initial findings they recommend further investigation with a larger, more diverse sample. Because of the negative relationship of lack of exercise, smoking, alcohol, and caffeine use on the general health and well-being of nursing students, Chow and Kalischuck (2008) investigated health-promotion and self-care behaviors of a group of 211 nursing students. They found that the majority of students did engage in some health-promoting self-care behaviors, and complementary alternative medicine (CAM). However, because of demanding schedules they often did not have enough time to sleep, eat, hydrate, and engage in self-care activities. Engaging in self-care activities has many positive benefits and can easily be incorporated into daily life. The key is to find the ones that you most enjoy and that provide you with the greatest benefits.

SELF-CARE STRATEGIES AND ACTIVITIES

There are so many ways to engage in self-care; it is advisable to try different activities until you find the ones that resonate with you. You are probably already engaging in some type of self-care activities and just need to incorporate them regularly into your daily life. The key is to select the things that you most enjoy because then you will be more likely to do them more frequently. "Self-care is the practice of health-related activities in which individuals engage in order to adopt a healthier lifestyle" (Lipson & Steiger, 1996, as cited in Stark & Manning-Walsh, 2005, p. 266). Stark and Manning-Walsh (2005) recommend preparing nursing students to engage in activities to promote healthy lifestyles while engaging in self-care, and further posit these activities should be learned in nursing schools so that students develop these strategies prior to their transition into professional practice. In their study on self-care they used a pre- and post-test approach on 66 nursing students to evaluate whether attendance at a mandatory class was related to self-care. They found that in general students did engage in the self-care activities of their choice after completing this class. Based on this study, Stark and Manning-Walsh (2005) recommend that self-care theory be included in the curriculum, and that students be given time in clinical practice to learn how to engage in self-care. They also recommend that future research be conducted with a larger, more diverse group of students. The results of these types of studies lend support to the premise that self-care is an important issue to include in the curriculum and throughout one's career as a nurse.

HOLISTIC NURSING PRACTICE

Holistic nursing is embedded in many nursing programs throughout the world and serves as a basis for many of the self-care strategies that will be discussed in this chapter.

Holistic nursing practice is guided by the holistic caring process, whether used with individuals, families, population groups, or communities. This process involves assessment, diagnosis, outcome identification, planning, implementation, and evaluation. It encompasses all significant actions taken in providing culturally and ethically respectful, compassionate, and relevant holistic nursing care to all persons (Mariano, 2006).

The underlying beliefs of holistic nursing practice are that health and illness are subjective and based on the individual's view. Therefore, it is imperative to involve the person in all aspects of care. Furthermore, "all people have an innate power and capacity for self-healing" (Mariano, 2006, p. 38). According to the Standards of Holistic Nursing Practice, "The nurse's self-reflection and self-assessment, self-care, healing, and personal development are necessary for service to others and growth/ change in one's own well-being and understanding of one's own personal journey. The nurse values oneself and one's calling to holistic nursing as a life purpose" (Mariano, 2006, p. 37).

There are many ways to engage in self-care, and in the next section an overview of some of the most common ones will be presented. Many of them fall under the umbrella of CAM, and have been practiced for many years. There are no right or wrong ways to do this, rather it is advantageous to experiment and choose the ones that you find most effective and beneficial (Raingruber & Robinson, 2007).

CONTEMPLATIVE PRACTICES

Contemplative practices are described as the various methods used as a means to quiet the mind and develop deep concentration. Examples of contemplative practices include all types of meditation, writing, contemplative arts, and movement. Contemplative practices help us to connect with things we find most meaningful and may help to reduce stress, improve communication and empathy, and enhance creativity and focus (The Center for Contemplative Mind in Society, 2013). Contemplative practices, such as yoga, meditation, and tai chi, have been effective in reducing stress and burnout in nurses (Raingruber & Robinson, 2007). Raingruber and Robinson (2007) conducted a qualitative study on 35 nurses to examine the effects of these self-care strategies, and concluded that these practices were related to a positive work environment, with nurses having greater focus and being more sensitive to patient's needs.

Some self-care strategies, such as deep breathing and meditation, can be done independently, whereas others, such as tai chi and reiki, require attendance at a formal program—at least initially to learn the basic concepts. Deep breathing and relaxation exercises are easy to do, can be done anywhere at any time, and are very helpful in promoting mindfulness and decreasing stress. Tai chi is an ancient Chinese martial art with a set of slowly paced and smoothly connected movements of all body parts. In tai chi one engages in gentle exercise, stretching, and deep breathing. It was originally developed as a form of self-defense, but is also used to treat many health conditions and may be helpful in decreasing stress (Mayo Clinic Staff, 2012). "Tai chi emphasizes mind–body connection during these movements" (Palumbo et al., 2012, p. 55). It has also been described as "meditation in motion" and because it involves gentle exercise most people can safely practice this ancient art (Mayo Clinic, 2012).

Many people find yoga to be an enjoyable and relaxing activity. "Yoga is an ancient discipline designed to bring balance and health to the physical, mental, emotional, and spiritual dimensions of the individual" (Ross & Thomas, 2010, p. 3). Yoga has become very popular in recent years and many studies have identified the positive benefits of this ancient practice (Ross & Thomas, 2010). For example, in their comprehensive review of the literature, Ross and Thomas (2010) found that yoga was related to positive health outcomes and subjective reports of pain, fatigue, and sleep. However, they do point out that future studies should be more rigorous and use larger, more diverse sampling. According to the American Yoga Association (2013), yoga is a practice that dates back over 5,000 years, when it was developed to promote harmony between the mind and body, and focuses on breathing, meditation, and exercise. In yoga the body is considered sacred, and the student must treat the body as a temple. The student initially engages in mindful exercise and control of one's breathing, breath being the source of life in the body. This helps to prepare the body for meditation, helps to clear the mind, and promotes healing. For best results one should engage in yoga on a daily basis. There are many types/forms of yoga and initially attending formal classes is beneficial. There are a myriad of books and DVDs that you may also wish to purchase or borrow from your public or school library. Once you learn the techniques you can incorporate them into your activities of daily living.

Meditation, deep-breathing, and relaxation are stress-reducing techniques that can be used alone or in conjunction with other types of self-care practices. "Meditation is a conscious mental process that induces a set of physiological changes termed as the relaxation response" (Huibing Lim et al., 2013, p. 12). It has been well documented that the nursing profession is quite stressful and may have a negative effect on the health and well-being of the nurse. Many studies have demonstrated the benefits of meditation in regards to stress reduction. However, according to Huibing Lim et al. (2013) these studies have been mainly done in Western countries. Huibing Lim et al. (2013) completed a review of the literature on meditation programs used by nurses. They examined eight studies that included mindfulness-based stress reduction (MBSR), eight-point program (EPP), mantra repetition program, and a computer-guided meditation program. They concluded that engaging in a mindful meditation program may reduce stress levels in nurses. Meditation can be done on an individual basis or in a group. Some people prefer to meditate in isolation, whereas others prefer a group setting. Initially you may need someone to guide you through some meditation exercises so that you can learn how to become centered and focused. In the beginning it is easy to become distracted by background sounds; however, once this becomes a part of your daily routine you will be able to block out all the noise and get into the "zone" whenever you feel the need to de-stress. There are books and DVDs that may be purchased if you prefer to meditate in the privacy of your home. You can even make up your own meditation tape or DVD using the meditation exercise below. You can edit the guide below to fit your own needs.

Meditation Exercise From Deborah Ann (Dr. Hunt)

Breathing is key. First, try to find a quiet and comfortable spot; you may play some spa/relaxing music, and light a lavender candle or lavender oil. I always recommend that you close your eyes and start with six slow, deep cleansing breaths while clearing your mind of all thoughts. Then with each additional breath on every exhalation concentrate on relaxing a body part. I usually start with my head and work down to my feet. Some people do it the other way. The key is to let yourself feel more relaxed with each exhalation. Like you are sinking into the chair or your bed or floating on a big white fluffy cloud. Then, when you are totally relaxed, continue to breathe slowly with your eyes closed and think about your favorite most relaxing place. It could be the beach, country, lake, or a favorite room in your house. I like to picture myself at the beach lying on the warm sand, smelling the fresh ocean air, and feeling the gentle breezes and warm rays of sun washing over me. Try to do this for at least 5 minutes and before you bring yourself back to reality, give yourself a positive thought, for example, "When I open my eyes I will feel refreshed." When you do this on a daily basis you will be amazed at how quickly you can put yourself into the "zone"— Happy Meditating.

There are many types of meditation, one example of which is *Sahaja* yoga meditation (Chung et al., 2012). In this type of meditation one engages in deep breathing and relaxation exercises while saying silent affirmations. Some individuals soak their feet in warm salt water while engaging in this type of meditation. When done daily, this practice has been associated with improved quality of life, decreased blood pressure, and decreased anxiety (Chung et al., 2012). Two other types of meditation that have been investigated are mindfulness meditation (MM), and transcendental meditation (TM). Breathing is central to the various meditations and in mindfulness meditation one engages in deep breathing and relaxation but does not suppress one's thoughts, rather one becomes more aware of these thoughts. Conversely, in transcendental meditation, one does not have a specific focus but does repeat a silent mantra while engaging in deep breathing and relaxation (Schoormans & Nyklí ček, 2011). The literature is replete with many different types of medication definitions and practices so it may take time before you find one model/technique that you prefer. Although many studies on the benefits of meditation have used different models, definitions, and techniques, there is a recognized relationship among meditation, stress reduction, and well-being (Huibing Lim et al., 2013; Schoormans & Nyklíček, 2011). According to Schoormans and Nyklíček (2011) there are several essential elements of meditation. For example, there should be a defined technique and a self-induced state occurs through mindful medication, in addition to an altered mode of consciousness.

There are many activities that you can engage in that have been associated with stress reduction and a feeling of well-being. Some of these include music therapy, art therapy, dancing, exercise, sports, physical activity, reading, and journaling. Basically any type of exercise will be beneficial; walking, jogging, aerobic exercise, dancing, sports programs, and strength training are some of the common ones. The benefits of art and music therapy, especially in stress reduction, have been widely discussed in the literature: painting, drawing, sculpting, and all types of music (Abbot et al., 2012; Lai & Li, 2011). Journaling, which will be further discussed in Chapter 16, has also been identified as a significant factor in stress reduction and coping (Thew, 2007). For example, Horneffer and Jamison (2002) found that journaling after a stressful event was related to greater improvement in emotional health, especially in male patients.

COMPLEMENTARY ALTERNATIVE MEDICINE

Complementary and alternative medicine is the umbrella term for health practices and beliefs that do not follow the biomedical model. Many of them are based on ancient healing modalities and Eastern philosophies. CAM is defined as a set of "diverse medical and health-care systems, practices, and products which are not considered a part of traditional medicine" (National Center for Complementary and Alternative Medicine [NCCAM], 2011, p. 1, as cited in Goldbas, 2012, p. 17). Many studies have been conducted on various CAM therapies and have found them to be effective in treating pain, and promoting health and well-being (Goldbas, 2012).
CAM includes:

- Acupuncture/acupressure—use of needles or pressure to specific parts of the body
- Herbal remedies—use of natural substances that are not U. S. Food and Drug Administration (FDA) approved and some that are not safe (for example, the following herbal remedies may be unsafe for pregnant women: chamomile, peppermint, ginger, and raspberry leaf [Wikinson, 2010]).
- Homeopathy—use of natural and toxic substances that are taken in very small doses; it high doses these substances can be fatal; it is best to consult a practitioner who specializes in homeopathy to restore balance in the body
- Mind–body techniques—including hypnosis and guided imagery
- Massage therapy—involves massaging of muscles and tissues
- Reiki—use of energy for healing
- Special diets—there are multiple types of diets and supplements that may aid in healing different conditions (Mayo Clinic, 2011)

It is important to have an understanding and basic knowledge of these practices as you may find them useful in maintaining balance and promoting self-healing. Furthermore, according to the Mayo Clinic (2011) 40% of the adult population currently engages in some type of CAM, and more and more health care practitioners are incorporating alternative therapies into their practice as an adjuvant to mainstream medical therapies. Even more interesting is the fact that 70% of people in the developing world and 91% of oncology patients in the United States use some form of CAM, which, in addition to what has previously been discussed, includes biofeedback, aromatherapy, cupping, spiritual healing and prayer, ayurvedic medicine, magnetic field therapy, and chiropractic medicine (Somani et al., 2014). Somani et al. (2014) found that although many nurses have a positive attitude about CAM, there is a lack of knowledge about CAM among nurses and therefore these types of modalities should be included in the nursing curricula. Although many of these practices are safe there may be potential adverse reactions between prescribed medications and herbal supplements (Mayo Clinic, 2011). As a nurse you are one of the prime patient advocates so it is important to understand these modalities for your own use and also in regard to your patients.

RESILIENCY

Resiliency is the ability to positively deal with stressful situations. People who are resilient can develop self-care strategies to cope with the continuing stress they face in their daily lives. Ahearn (2006), states, "The concept of resilience has been commonly referred to as the ability to "spring back" and is similarly defined in research and clinical practice" (p. 1). Resiliency definitions have two essential attributes, "(1) 'good' or positive outcomes that occur in spite of (2) adverse conditions" (Masten, 2001, as cited in Peterson & Bredow, 2004, p. 344).

There have been several studies that have investigated the relationship of resiliency, stress, and burnout. Some researchers believe that if nurses, especially new graduate nurses, are educated on resilience and are taught ways to improve personal resilience there will be decreased stress and burnout (Hodges & Grier, 2004; Pines et al. 2012). Burnout is defined as "a syndrome of emotional exhaustion and cynicism that occurs frequently among individuals who do "people work" of some kind" (Toscano, 1998). Several studies have been undertaken on resiliency in relation to nursing education and nursing service. For example, Edward (2005) completed a study on the phenomenon of resilience in mental health clinicians. The study was composed of six participants who were crisis care clinicians in mental health. Resilience in this study was defined as "the ability of an individual to bounce back from adversity and persevere through difficult times" (p. 152). The participants were interviewed and identified descriptions related to resiliency, such as "the team is a protective veneer to the stress of work; having a sense of self; faith and hope; having insight; and looking after self." The study addressed mental health and the positive effect that resilience may have on burnout, turnover rates and retention. The study, although limited, demonstrated a link between resilience and retention. The study did not address how to develop personal resiliency but did show the traits of resiliency and the potential positive effects in improving retention. Hodges, Keeley, and Grier (2004) discuss resilience and Parse's theory of human science as a way to improve the retention of new nurses. Resilience is a vital trait that can be learned and can foster growth and opportunity in response to adversity. Using Parse's theoretical framework can guide nurse educators in fostering the development of resilience in nursing students. Student–faculty dyads can be used to identify philosophies of caring and develop professional identities. A study by Jacelon (2004) was undertaken on resilience in regard to it being a trait or a process. The purpose of this study was to review the literature on resilience as an inherent trait versus a process. Resilience as a trait was defined by Wagnild and Young (1993) as "a personality characteristic that moderates the negative effects of stress and promotes adaptation" (p. 165). This type of resilience has become inherent in the person and may have been influenced by past experience and intellectual ability. Flach (1980) described the dynamic process of resiliency as "a system which can be learned at any point in life" (as cited in Jacelon, 2004, p. 128). Hodges and Grier (2004) addressed the concept of using Parse's human science theory as a theoretical framework for nursing education as well as "a framework with which to promote professional resilience and career longevity by purposefully engaging students within student–faculty dyads to explore personal meanings and philosophies of caring, and to create strong professional identities" (p. 548). The authors of this study made a strong connection to the role of academic education in laying the foundation for a nurse to be successful and have longevity. Using Parse's theory as a framework in nursing education could have a positive impact on the future of nurses. At the very least the part about resiliency can be incorporated into any framework. A school then could partner with a hospital where continued development of resilience, mentoring and education could be incorporated. "Educators can emphasize skills that focus on solutions, rather than problems, on building resilience and professional stamina" (Hodge, Keely and Grier, 2004, p. 550). Nursing students face many challenges and adversity throughout nursing school and Hodge et al. (2008) suggest that new nurses must find a way to thrive, especially in a tumultuous acute care setting. "Nurse educators must design pedagogies that address professional socialization and the development of resilience behaviors in the educational setting that will facilitate safe passage through the tumultuous times of the first 18 months of practice" (Hodge et al., 2008, p. 88). Pines et al. (2012) found a relationship among empowerment, stress resiliency, and conflict management. "Stress resiliency and psychological empowerment are human traits, combining to strengthen the capacity of an individual to respond to stressors" (Pines et al., 2012, p. 1483). Although it is a well-known fact that some people are more resilient than others recent studies have supported the premise that resiliency can be increased. For example, Moran (2012) posits "Graduate nurses can also become more resilient through learned coping behavior" (p. 273). Developing coping strategies and engaging in self-care activities are two ways nurses can increase their resiliency (Moran, 2012).

The United Kingdom has recently developed a Care campaign in an effort to improve patient care and one of the initiatives is to build resiliency in nurses. Citing issues of anxiety, stress, and burnout among nurses and the implications for poor patient care, a comprehensive initiative has been developed. Strategies that are aimed at building resiliency include improving work environments, administrative support, and stress reduction (Dean, 2012). Another factor that relates to resiliency is hardiness, which refers to having the ability to deal positively with a stressful situation. "Findings have shown that hardiness enhances resiliency in a wide range of stressful circumstances" (Maddi, 2005, p. 261). It is well known that resiliency varies among individuals and the literature is replete with information on the significance of resilience in patients and nurses. There are many wonderful resources and online assessment tools you can use to assess your level of resiliency and engage in activities that will increase your level or resiliency.

You can complete a quiz on your resiliency at the following website:http://psychology.about.com/library/quiz/blresiliencea.htm

SELF-ADVOCACY

Advocacy is an important concept in nursing and most often this term is used in reference to the patient. A patient advocate is defined as "someone who defends the patient against 'infringements of his or her rights" (Winslow, 1984, as cited in Mahlin, 2010, p. 248). A more specific definition in relation to the nursing profession is "the nurse is to actively support patients in speaking up for their rights and choices, in helping patients to clarify their decisions, in furthering their legitimate interests, and protecting their basic rights as persons, such as privacy and autonomy in decision making" (Hamrac, 2000, as cited in Mahlin, 2010, p. 248). Self-advocacy is a matter of acting on one's own behalf, either as a member of society in general or in a particular arena. Although it may be challenging to advocate for one's self it is extremely important, especially in nursing. Advocacy will be the mainstay of your life; first as a student and then throughout your professional career. You will need to learn how to be a patient advocate in addition to learning how to advocate for yourself. Being able to advocate for yourself will be invaluable as you complete your journey into the world of nursing. For example, there may be times when the challenges of your program are very overwhelming and it will be important to be able to explore options that will foster success. As a college student you will need to know how to advocate for yourself because you are now an adult learner. It is very important to be proactive. Therefore, if you are not doing well in a particular course you need to meet with your instructor to discuss strategies and ways to be successful. This could involve the use of a tutor, study groups, or one-on-one consultation with your instructor. Furthermore, you may need to request an "incomplete" or "withdraw" from the course. These options, although sometimes the best course of action, have specific requirements and deadlines. You cannot wait until the end of the semester to start advocating for yourself. You always need to take a proactive approach. Believe it or not, most faculty are very understanding and will try to work with you as long as academic integrity is not compromised or school policy violated. Sometimes even the most organized and high-achieving students fall behind in their studies due to circumstances beyond their control. If you need an extension for an assignment you should contact your instructor as early as possible to discuss options. Don't wait until the day something is due to ask for an extension. Remember, procrastination will not help you be successful. This is also true of your future role as a professional nurse. For example, you will need to advocate for yourself as you transition into your profession. Communicating your learning needs to your preceptor and manager will be extremely important. Attending formal classes that teach self-awareness and communication can help one become more assertive and build on self-esteem (Ünal, 2012), which may help in the development of self-advocacy skills. Learning how to engage in self-advocacy will require persistence, perseverance, courage, and belief in yourself. Although, initially it may be a difficult task it will be well worth the effort.

TOP 10 TIPS FOR SELF-CARE AND RESILIENCY

1. Complete a self-assessment of your self-care and resiliency.
2. Get enough rest.
3. Eat healthily.
4. Don't smoke.
5. Improve communication skills.
6. Find a mentor.
7. Role play.
8. Believe in yourself.
9. Engage in self-care and stress reduction activities.
10. Seek ways to develop coping skills.

SUMMARY

This chapter focused on the importance of engaging in self-care, resiliency development, and advocacy. An overview of various self-care strategies was provided in addition to a sample meditation exercise and a link to an online resiliency quiz.

DISCUSSION QUESTIONS

1. Discuss some of the challenges faced by student nurses.
2. What are some of the negative effects of stress?
3. Discuss burnout and how it relates to nursing students and nurses.
4. Discuss the importance of self-care as a student and a nurse.
5. List and describe at least five self-care strategies.
6. What is holistic nursing?
7. Discuss the unique aspects of complementary and alternative medicine.
8. List and discuss three types of CAM.
9. Discuss resiliency and ways to become more resilient.
10. Discuss the significance of advocacy and self-advocacy in relation to students and nurses.

SUGGESTED LEARNING ACTIVITIES

- Complete a self-assessment on resiliency.
- Practice the meditation exercise on p 39.
- Engage in at least one self-care activity discussed in this chapter.
- Conduct a literature review on the use of CAM and write a three-page essay.
- Start a support group at your school.
- Interview a nurse, a faculty member, and a fellow student about their resiliency and self-care strategies.

REFERENCES

Abbott, K. A., Shanahan, M. J., & Nuefield, J. (2013). Artistic tasks outperform nonartistic tasks for stress reduction. *Art Therapy: Journal of the American Art Therapy Association, 30*(2), 71–78.

Ahearn, N. R. (2006). Adolescent Resilience: An evolutionary concept analysis. *Journal of Pediatric Nursing, 21*(3), 1–22.

Aiken, L. H., Clarke, S. P., Sochalski, J. H., & Silber, J. H. (n.d.). Hospital nurse staffing and patient mortality, nurse burnout and job dissatisfaction. *Journal for American Medical Association, 288*(16), 1987–1994.

American Yoga Association. (2013). *General information.* Retrieved from www.americanyogaassociation.org/contents.html

Block, L. M., Claffey, C., Korow, M. C., & McCaffery, R. (2005). The value of mentorship within nursing organizations. *Nursing Forum, 40*(4), 134–140.

The Center for Contemplative Mind in Society. (2013). *Contemplative practices.* Retrieved from https://www.contemplativemind.org/practices

Chow, J., & Kalischuk, R. (2008). Self-care for caring practice: Student nurses' perspectives. *International Journal For Human Caring, 12*(3), 31–37.

Chung, S., Brooks, M. M., Rai, M., Balk, J. L., & Rai, S. (2012). Effect of Sahaja yoga meditation on quality of life, anxiety, and blood pressure Control. *Journal of Alternative & Complementary Medicine, 18*(6), 589–596. doi:10.1089/acm.2011.0038

Complementary and alternative medicine in oncology nursing. (2014). *British Journal of Nursing, 23*(1), 40–46.

Cook, K. (n.d.). The heartbeat of healthcare battles burnout. *Arizona Nurse, 59*(3), 11.

Daly, J., Chang, E., & Jackson, D. (2006). Quality of work life in nursing: Some issues and challenges. *Collegian, 13*(4), 1–3.

Dean, E. (2012). Building resilience. *Nursing Standard, 26*(32), 16–18.

Edward, K. L. (2005). The Phenomenon of resilience in crisis care mental health clinicians. *International Journal of Mental Health, 14*(2), 142–148.

Goldbas, A. (2012). An introduction to complementary and alternative medicine (CAM). *International Journal of Childbirth Education, 27*(3), 16–20.

Gould, D. (2005). Return-to-practice initiatives in nursing retention. *Nursing Standard Online, 19*(47), 41–46.

Hinshaw, A. S., Smeltzer, C.H., & Atwood, J.R. (1987). Innovative retention strategies for nursing staff. *Journal of Nursing Administration, 17*(6), 8–16.

Hodges, H.F., Keeley, A.C., & Grier, E.E. (2004). Professional resilience, practice longevity, and Parse's theory for baccalaureate education. *Journal of Nursing Education, 44*(12), 548–554.

Horneffer, K., & Jamison, P. (2002). The emotional effects of writing about stressful experiences: An exploration of moderators. *Occupational Therapy in Health Care, 16*(2/3), 77–89.

Huibing Lim, M., Chow Yeow, L., & Poon, E. (2013). Evaluation of meditation programmes used by nurses to reduce stress: A literature review. *Singapore Nursing Journal, 40*(3), 11–20.

Jacelon, C. S. (1997). The trait and process of resilience. *Journal of Advanced Nursing, 25,* 123–129.

Kravitz, K., McAllister-Black, R., Grant, M., & Kirk, C. (2010). Self-care strategies for nurses: A psycho-educational intervention for stress reduction and the prevention of burnout. *Applied Nursing Research, 23*(3), 130–138. doi:10.1016/j.apnr.2008.08.002

Lai, H., & Li, Y. (2011). The effect of music on biochemical markers and self-perceived stress among first-line nurses: A randomized controlled crossover trial. *Journal of Advanced Nursing, 67*(11),

Laschinger, H. K., & Wong, C. A. (2006). The impact of staff nurse empowerment on person–job fit and work engagement/burnout. *Nurse Administration Quarterly, 30*(4), 358–367.

Lusler, K. G. (2006). Recruitment & retention report: Taming burnout's flame. *Nursing Management, 37*(4), 14.

Maddi, S. (2005). On hardiness and other pathways to resilience. *American Psychologist, 60*(3), 261–272.

Mahlin, M. (2010). Individual patient advocacy, collective responsibility and activism within professional nursing associations. *Nursing Ethics 17*(2) 247–254.

Mariano, C. (2006). *Holistic nursing: Scope and standards of practice.* New York, NY: American Nurses Association.

Mayo Clinic Staff. (2011). *Complementary and alternative medicine.* Retrieved from https://www.mayoclinic.com/health/alternative-medicine/PN00001

Mayo Clinic Staff. (2012). *Tai chi: A gentle way to fight stress.* Retrieved from https://www.mayoclinic.com/health/tai-chi/SA00087

McCarthy, P. (1986). A wellness program for student nurses: Studying its effects on health values, health locus of control, and self-care agency. *Journal of Holistic Nursing, 4*(1), 31–34.

Moran, R. (2012). Retention of new graduate nurses: The literature informs staff educators [online serial]. *Journal for Nurses in Staff Development* [serial online], *28*(6), 270–273. doi: 10.1097/NND.0b013e318272584a.

National Center for Complementary and Alternative Medicine. (2011). *What is complementary and alternative medicine?* Retrieved from http://www.nccam.nih.gov/health/whatiscam

The New York Academy for Medicine & Jonas Center for Nursing Excellence. (2006). *Nurse retention and workforce diversity—Two key issues in New York City's nursing crisis.* Retrieved from http://www.nyam.org/search.jsp?query=Jonas+Center&x=0&y=0

Nursing theories—Orem's self-care nursing theory. (2012). Retrieved from http://currentnursing.com/nursing_theory/self_care_deficit_theory.html

Orem, D. (1995). *Nursing: Concepts of practice.* St. Louis, MO: Mosby

Palumbo, M., Wu, G., Shaner-McRae, H., Rambur, B., & McIntosh, B. (2012). Tai Chi for older nurses: A workplace wellness pilot study. *Applied Nursing Research, 25*(1), 54–59. doi:10.1016/j.apnr.2010.01.002

Peterson, S., & Bredow, T. (2004). *Middle range theories: Application to nursing research.* Philadelphia: Lippincott, Williams & Wilkinson.

Pines, E. W., Rauschhuber, M. L., Norgan, G. H., Cook, J. D., Canchola, L., Richardson, C., & Jones, M. (2012). Stress resiliency, psychological empowerment and conflict management styles among baccalaureate nursing students. *Journal of Advanced Nursing, 68*(7), 1482–1493. doi:10.1111/j.1365-2648.2011.05875.x

Raingruber, B., & Robinson, C. (2007). The effectiveness of tai chi, yoga, meditation, and Reiki healing sessions in promoting health and enhancing problem solving abilities of registered nurses. *Issues in Mental Health Nursing, 28*(10), 1141–1155.

Ranheim, A., Kärner, A., & Berterö, C. (2012). Caring theory and practice—Entering a simultaneous concept analysis. *Nursing Forum, 47*(2), 78–90. doi:10.1111/j.1744-6198.2012.00263.x

Ross, A., & Thomas, S. (2010). The health benefits of yoga and exercise: A review of comparison studies. *Journal of Alternative & Complementary Medicine, 16*(1), 3-12. doi:10.1089/acm.2009.0044

Schoormans, D., & Nyklíček, I. (2011). Mindfulness and psychologic well-being: Are they related to type of meditation technique practiced? *Journal of Alternative & Complementary Medicine, 17*(7), 629–634. doi:10.1089/acm.2010.0332

Siebert, A. (n.d.). *How to develop resiliency strengths.* Retrieved from https://www.resiliencycenter.com

Somani S., Ali F., Saeed Ali T., Sulaiman Lailani, N. (2014). Complementary and alternative medicine in oncology nursing. *British Journal of Nursing, 23*(1), 40-46.

Stark, M., Manning-Walsh, J., & Vliem, S. (2005). Caring for self while learning to care for others: A challenge for nursing students. *Journal of Nursing Education, 44*(6), 266–270.

Thew, J. (2007). Tune into your surroundings: The practice of art journaling can provide an outlet for health professionals to express emotion and to reflect. *Nursing Spectrum (Midwest), 8*(10), 12–13.

Toscano, P., & Pointerdolph, M. (1998). The personality to buffer burnout. *Nursing Management, 29*(8):32L, 32N, 32R.

Trossman, S. (2013). A study in de-stressing. (Cover story). *American Nurse, 45*(3), 1–11.

Ünal, S. (2012). Evaluating the effect of self-awareness and communication techniques on nurses' assertiveness and self-esteem. *Contemporary Nurse: A Journal for the Australian Nursing Profession, 43*(1), 90–98. doi:10.5172/conu.2012.43.1.90

Wagnild, G. M., & Young, H. M. (1993). Development and psychometric evaluation of the resilience scale. *Journal of Nursing Measurement, 1,* 165–178. Retrieved from https://www.resiliencescale.com

Watson, J. (1988). *Nursing: Human science and human care—A theory of nursing.* New York, NY: National League for Nursing.

Watson, J. (2008). *Nursing: The philosophy and science of caring* (rev. ed.). Boulder, CO: University Press of Colorado.

Wilkinson, J. (2000). What do we know about herbal morning sickness treatments? A literature survey. *Midwifery, 16*(3), 224–228.

CHAPTER 4

Portfolio Development

A mind that is stretched by a new experience can never go back to its old dimensions.

—Oliver Wendell Holmes, Jr.

OBJECTIVES

After reading this chapter, the reader will be able to:

- Understand the difference between a student and professional portfolio
- Discuss the importance of a portfolio
- Develop a professional portfolio
- Identify the key information to include in a portfolio
- Explore various portfolio development programs.

Portfolios have been used for many years, especially in the world of art and business (Timmins & Dunne, 2009). Currently, portfolios are used both academically and professionally and are embraced by many disciplines around the world (Nairn et al., 2006). The use of portfolios in nursing education has become very popular in recent years (Nairn et al., 2006). A portfolio is basically a snapshot of accomplishments as a student or a professional. The portfolio is tailored to and developed based on specific use: academic studies or profession. For example, art students develop a portfolio of their artwork to demonstrate their accomplishments and share their work. According to Casey and Egan (2010), the professional portfolio should "provide evidence of how an individual has developed both personally and professionally. It is therefore a showcase for past accomplishments and achievements, but can also be used as a dynamic vehicle to enable future career and development planning" (p. 547). This chapter focuses on both academic and professional portfolios. It includes valuable information about how to develop a portfolio as a student and a professional, and the importance of updating it throughout your entire career. Although portfolio development is done on an individual basis and each one is unique to its owner there are some commonalities, such as the inclusion of your résumé/curriculum vita and supporting documents. Portfolios will also vary based on their intended purpose. For example, academic portfolios may be developed for a course requirement with specific learning objectives and guidelines. Professional portfolios will be developed to demonstrate your experience and accomplishments when applying for a position or promotion. Whether for academic or professional use, similar to résumés/curriculum vitaes, portfolios need to be of high quality and updated on a continual basis.

THE PORTFOLIO

The term "portfolio" has many different meanings. It may defined as a case for carrying documents or as the collected investment holdings of an individual or institution.

The portfolio you develop as a student, and later as a professional nurse, will be somewhat different than the ones described above. Of course, you may choose to use a flat, portable case, but the contents will be different. However, it is much more likely that you will develop an e-portfolio as it will be much easier to update and share. Furthermore, the Internet is replete with programs, some free and some for a fee, that provide templates and guidelines for developing an e-portfolio. In this age of ever-expanding technology, an e-portfolio is the better option. Indeed some schools subscribe to a service so that all students use the same program. In support of this in a study comparing web- and paper-based portfolio development, Driessen et al. (2009) found that the use of web-based portfolios increased student motivation and that faculty found them to be easier to use. Interestingly, there was no difference in the quality of either type of portfolio; however, because of student and faculty motivation the web-based version may be the better option.

ACADEMIC AND STUDENT PORTFOLIOS

Portfolios have a multitude of uses and applications in the academic setting. For example, they are used to demonstrate students' academic and professional achievements, and are currently being used across the curriculum (Nairn et al., 2006). Academic portfolios have become increasingly popular among nursing faculty and are now being incorporated into various courses as a means of teaching and assessment (Nairn et al., 2006). According to Nairn et al. (2006), "The main purpose of developing a portfolio is to link understanding about clinical experiences and theoretical knowledge within a discipline" (p. 1510). It has also been viewed as a way to address the theory–practice gap commonly observed in nursing students, and it helps the student to become actively involved in their learning (Nairn et al., 2006). As an adult learner the onus will be on the student to be a self-directed learner. However, despite being an adult learner some students require more guidance and assistance than others. Initially, engaging in portfolio development can be somewhat daunting and students may not appreciate the significance of this activity. Interestingly, Davis et al. (2009) found that although students believed that the "paperwork was excessive" at the end of the 4 years students became more positive about portfolio development (p. 89).

When used in a formal manner for a specific course or program of study you will most likely be provided with specific course objectives and guidelines for completion. Even though you may be developing a course-specific portfolio it will be quite easy to revise and edit it so it can be used as your professional portfolio upon graduation. Portfolios may be used to evaluate student outcomes and assess a student's ability to achieve the desired level of competency in communication and problem-solving, as well as the ability to critically think and reason (Rossetti et al., 2012). An example of the use of student portfolios in an undergraduate nursing program proved to be very successful. A committee of faculty and students collaborated on the process using clear guidelines, objectives, and rubrics. Freshmen were provided with an orientation about the use of portfolios but did not begin the formal development until their third semester. Rossetti et al. (2012) shared the following example of a student portfolio. The portfolio required a cover letter that reflected on their selected assignments in relation to the required outcomes of writing, critical thinking, and therapeutic interventions.

Students were also asked to complete a self-evaluation and reflect on the process. Self-evaluation is considered a critical step in portfolio development. Rossetti et al. (2012) concluded that the use of portfolios was viewed positively, and although there are still some issues with students writing ability and use of APA (American Psychological Association) style the faculty have noted improvements. Clearly, there has been progress in the use and value of portfolios because in an earlier study by Williams et al. (2009) students became less enthused about the use of portfolios as they progressed to senior level, with some seeing them as a time-consuming exercise without clear benefits. Williams et al. (2009) also point out that very few professional nurses use portfolios, which may cause students to question their value.

McMullan et al. (2003) completed a review of the literature and concluded that portfolios are indeed a valid way to assess student outcomes and competency achievement. Evaluating students' competencies and learning outcomes can be challenging, and the use of portfolios provides a holistic way to evaluate student outcomes. However, there are important components that must be included when using a portfolio for student assessment. First and foremost there should be specific guidelines for the portfolio program that are based on sound theoretical concepts. There must also be student reflection on the process and collaboration between the faculty and students. Furthermore, the portfolio program should be reassessed and revised on a continual basis. "In summary, a portfolio is a collection of evidence, usually in written form, of both the products and processes of learning. It attests to achievement and personal and professional development, by providing critical analysis of its contents" (McMullen et al., 2003, p. 288). As a student you will want to take this assignment quite seriously as a well-developed portfolio will help you to identify your strengths and weaknesses. It will also provide you, your faculty, and future employers with objective evidence of your accomplishments. All students have different strengths and weaknesses, and potential. Developing a comprehensive and quality portfolio can help you to identify all of these things, which in turn can be used for self-improvement. Self-evaluation is one of the hardest things you will encounter, but it is very important. Portfolios provide a means to more objectively complete a self-evaluation. For example, when reviewing the documents you have included in your portfolio you can compare different items to see whether you have improved. You might compare a paper you wrote as a sophomore and a paper you wrote as a junior. It is to be hoped that the paper you wrote as a junior will be significantly improved, with evidence of scholarly writing, critical appraisal, and correct use of APA. However, if your paper is the same or worse, then you need to critically examine your actions and ponder the reasons for this. Perhaps, you were just rushed and did not devote adequate time. On the other hand, you may need to seek assistance from a writing tutor or spend time in the writing center at your school. Perhaps, you didn't understand the assignment and should have consulted with the faculty member before completing it. There are myriad reasons for doing poorly on an assignment, and scholarly writing can be particularly challenging. Your faculty understands scholarly writing is challenging, and that your early writings may not be perfect. However, as you progress through the academic program you should be able to demonstrate significant improvements in your academic achievements and scholarly writing.

One common issue with portfolio development is the lack of clear guidelines provided to students by their faculty. Furthermore, there appears to be limited evidence as to best practices in regard to portfolio use in the academic setting (Timmins & Dunne 2008). Although there are often no uniform or standard guidelines, many faculty do provide guidelines and if they don't you should consult them for clarification and guidance. There are three general types of portfolios. The first one is biographical and is often used by professional nurses. This type of portfolio includes a list of accomplishments: a résumé, educational achievements, awards, and honors. The second type is the learning portfolio, which is used in academic settings and may have specific learning objectives. The third type of portfolio is competency based, which is used to assess student competence and learning outcomes (Timmins & Dunne, 2008). The portfolio may be an actual assignment that will be graded and count toward your course grade. On the other hand, although it will be a formal assignment it may not be graded; however, even if it is not formally graded it will certainly be to your benefit to develop a perfect portfolio. All students, whether required or not, should begin compiling a portfolio as soon as possible. The years go by quickly and are faced with multiple obligations and, believe it or not, by the time you are a senior you may not remember the things you achieved as a freshman. Furthermore, it may be difficult to locate the various supporting documents you will need for your portfolio. Some schools have their students begin their portfolios during the first semester, whereas others wait until the student begins to complete the core course requirements related to the intended major. Some schools will not have any policies regarding portfolios and leave it up to the individual student to decide whether a portfolio will be beneficial.

In summary, the benefits of portfolios have been well documented and whether you develop one in fulfillment of a course requirement or not, you should give some serious thought to developing a professional portfolio before you graduate. This way it will be very easy to update as you transition into professional practice and eventually continue your educational journey toward a higher degree.

PROFESSIONAL PORTFOLIOS

Professional portfolios are similar to but different from academic portfolios. Academic portfolios, if completed for a specific assignment, may only have some of the items you will need for your professional portfolio. However, it is fairly easy to revise and update your academic portfolio. Remember this is a work in progress and will be used throughout your professional and academic journey to demonstrate your achievements. Portfolios may actually influence development and foster lifelong learning. Furthermore, they can be used to assess skills in the affective, cognitive, and reflective domains (Green et al., 2014)

The structure and presentation of a portfolio will clearly vary according to the individual's preferences, experiences, and career goals, but some common information and documentation to consider for inclusion are outlined below:

- Biographical information
- Educational background
- Employment history with brief description of roles and responsibilities
- Professional qualification certificates (Casey & Egan, 2010, p. 547)

The professional portfolio should demonstrate your development as a professional nurse. Basically, you want to show how you have gained knowledge and experience along your career trajectory. Although your résumé will include the information stated above, the portfolio will show how you have developed and improved throughout the years. Therefore, it is important to include documents that will support your statements and achievements. For example, if you receive an award for a particular accomplishment, in addition to including it on your résumé, you would also place a copy of the award in your portfolio.

Portfolios can be used to show competence in a particular area. Many nurses specialize in a particular area and eventually earn certification in their specialty. Most often this requires completion of a review course, successful completion of a national exam, and completion of a certain amount of continuing education credits to maintain certification. A portfolio is a tool developed by the registered professional nurse to provide evidence of achievements, knowledge, and attitudes. The portfolio is an individualized collection of materials that "reflect current development and activity of that individual" (Byrne et al., 2007, p. 26). Because the portfolio is a reflection of you it should be clearly organized and well developed. You should give careful thought and consideration as to what materials you will include in your portfolio. Although you want to present it in a holistic manner you need to do so in an orderly fashion. You don't want to include everything you ever did. Keep in mind that this portfolio will be read by others: colleagues, managers, or recruiters. According to Oermann (2002) there are two types of professional portfolios: "Best-work portfolios provide evidence of the nurse's competencies and expertise" (Oermann, 2002, p. 73). This type of well-organized portfolio is used to demonstrate competence and may be used for annual reviews, clinical ladders, or when applying for a new position. "Growth and development portfolios are designed for nurses to measure their progress in meeting personal and professional learning goals" (Oermann, 2002, pp. 73–74). The purpose of this type of portfolio is to demonstrate ongoing evidence of competencies. Documents to include in this type of portfolio are evidence of continuing education, competency evaluations, and annual appraisals. Oermann (2002) outlines a plan for developing a portfolio for professional development that includes the following steps:

1. Complete a learning needs assessment of self.
2. Develop a plan to meet learning needs identified in step 1.
3. Implement the plan (e.g., completing a certification course).
4. Evaluate your plan and validate completion of goals and objectives.

Oermann (2002) likens this to the nursing process, which involves assessment, planning, interventions, and evaluation and revision of the plan as needed. This is a wonderful way to demonstrate your achievements and your commitment to your professional development.

Some countries require portfolios when renewing licenses and/or recertification. For example, nurses in England (Oermann, 2002), Australia, and New Zealand must develop a portfolio that demonstrates their assessment of practice, current practice, and professional development (Sinclair et al., 2013). Continued professional development (CPD) is expected of every nurse in Australia and New Zealand. Each country has different guidelines for the amount and type of activity required. Activities include writing for publication, attending continuing education classes, presenting at workshops, working with a mentor, participating in research, and obtaining an advanced degree. Developing a plan that includes specific target dates, with measurable goals and objectives, along with a plan for evaluation and self-reflection is an important component of portfolio development (Sinclair et al., 2013). Similarly, Byrne et al. (2007) recommend creating a plan and rationale for developing your portfolio and selecting the documents. This will be further discussed in the next section.

PORTFOLIO DEVELOPMENT

Developing a portfolio is a formal process that requires careful planning and great attention to detail. Joyce (2005) used an action research approach to examine portfolio development by postgraduate nursing students, and identify a framework to guide the implementation of this type of portfolio. The emerging framework included professional development planning, tutors—academic and professional—and action-learning tutorials (Joyce, 2005). Although this framework focused on graduate nurses it is can also be used for personal-development planning and in the development of clinical career pathways (Joyce, 2005). A framework for portfolio development is a rather new concept, and clearly further research is warranted to identify best practices and models.

Before you begin your portfolio you need to consider whether you will be developing an academic or professional portfolio. Next you will need to decide whether you will develop an electronic portfolio or a hard copy, although you may not have a choice, especially if you are developing an academic portfolio. Even if you are not completing an online portfolio you should try to have as many of your documents on the computer as possible so they can be easily updated and accessed. Based on the type of portfolio you will then need to devise a plan for development. An academic portfolio will often have specific guidelines, although this is not always the case. However, if there are guidelines, then you should be sure to follow them exactly as stated. If you are developing a professional portfolio you will have to decide what to include and how you want to proceed. Keep in mind that this should be about quality not quantity. You may be tempted to put in everything but the kitchen sink but this will not be to your benefit, and it may actually have a negative effect. According to Hawks (2014), you should have a clear rationale for every document you place in your portfolio and should also evaluate all the documents you do include and reflect on whether or not they belong. Intuitively you might believe that you should only include exemplary papers and projects; however, if you want to demonstrate development and improvement it is probably best to include some "not so perfect" papers too, especially if this is an academic portfolio. This is a perfect way to demonstrate your growth and development over a period of time and shows not only your potential for future growth, but your actual growth. Developing a plan for your portfolio, whether hard copy or electronic, is a key component. If you prefer to use an electronic program and you are completing a student portfolio you should check with your school as they may already have one for you to use. There are many free programs offered online; some require a nominal fee. The templates, samples, and instructions that are often available with these programs are an added benefit to their use. Electronic portfolios are becoming more and more popular within the world of nursing. Although developing an online portfolio may seem like a daunting task to some, it certainly provides a valid way for one to document achievements, professional development, and ongoing learning (Green et al., 2014). Electronic portfolios allow you to provide a retrospective and prospective development and achievement of competencies (Hawks, 2014). Another benefit of electronic portfolios is that you can include a variety of evidence. According to Hawks (2014), electronic portfolios can include traditional items such as documents and certificates, and nontraditional items such as hyperlinks, images, blog entries, and electronic files. Thompson (2011) posits, "Many newer systems can upload continuing education attended within the health care system directly into the individual's portfolio and then directly to his/her résumé or curriculum vitae" (p. 170). Electronic portfolios are easy to maintain and update, and only take up a small amount of space on your computer. They are also easy to share with faculty, recruiters, and managers.

Although the electronic portfolio seems to be the preferred method, if you prefer to develop a hard copy version you should invest in a good-quality binder in a basic color like blue, black, or white. The size will depend on the type of portfolio and what you plan to include in it. Clearly you don't want to buy a small binder and overstuff it with documents. You also want to avoid a large binder that looks sparse because you are just beginning your academic or professional journey. You will also need to purchase labels and dividers. In general it is best to use a good-quality beige or white paper. Most people place the original copies of their documents in the binder, but it is important to make duplicate copies and keep them in a safe place. The key is to develop a binder that is neatly organized and maintained. You can always purchase a bigger binder as you advance in your academic and professional journey.

Although this is an individual task it is a good idea to have one or two experts review your portfolio, whether it is a hard copy or electronic version. This is an important compilation of your achievements and it must be practically perfect in every way. It can be difficult to judge your own work so having input can prove to be invaluable. Even if you cannot locate an expert you may request that your mentor, or at the very least a friend or family member, review it. The important thing is to elicit a nonbiased critique of your work. It can be difficult to hear negative comments; however, these should be viewed as constructive criticisms that will be quite beneficial.

Once you develop a portfolio you will want to reflect on it. Is it clearly written and error free? Is it well organized and neat? Did you include a table of contents? Did you clearly state your goals and objectives? Are the objectives and/or learning outcomes achievable and measurable? Have you included a well-developed résumé or curriculum vitae? Have you included valid and appropriate evidence of your achievements? Have you revised or updated your portfolio? Do you have a plan for how often you will review and update it? It is crucial to remember to continually update and expand on your portfolio.

Similar to your résumé your portfolio will be a work in progress and will need to be updated and revised throughout your academic and professional journey. You may have developed an exemplary portfolio in nursing school but once you embark on your professional journey you will need to revise your portfolio (see Tables 4.1 and 4.2). Although some of the contents will be applicable you want to demonstrate that you put a considerable amount of thought and effort into your portfolio. Remember, it is a reflection of your personal and professional achievements and will be viewed by various nurses, nurse educators, recruiters, and administrators. A well-developed portfolio speaks volumes and, similar to the résumé, is often the first impression you will make on recruiters and managers.

TABLE 4.1
Template/Example of a Professional Portfolio*

Welcome Page	First Page
Table of Contents	Second Page
• Professional Résumé	Section 1
• Self-Evaluation	
• Professional Development Plan	
• Goals and Objectives	Section 2
• Supporting Documents	Section 3

(continued)

TABLE 4.1
**Template/Example of a Professional Portfolio* *(continued)*

-Seminars

-Continuing Education

-Awards*

- Presentations*

-Publications*

-Peer Review

-Letters of Recommendation

-Diplomas

-Other

• Self-Reflection	Section 4

*If using an electronic journal you can place links to presentations, journals, and documents.

TABLE 4.2
Template/Example of an Academic Portfolio

Welcome Page	First Page
Table of Contents	Second Page
• Professional Résumé	Section 1
• Self-Evaluation	
• Competency Statement	
• Goals and Objectives	Section 2
• Lifelong Learning Activities	
• Supporting Documents	Section 3
-Scholarly Papers	
-Evaluations	
-Letters of Recommendation	
-Evidence of Achievement of Bachelor of Science in Nursing	
Competencies	
-Special Projects	
-Professional/Academic Activities	
-Honors and Awards	
-Professional Organizations	
• Self–Reflection	Section 4

Note: This is an example; follow the guidelines given by your school and/or instructor.

You should also include a reflective statement for your portfolio with a list of supporting documentation. You can upload papers, presentations, case studies, and so on that illustrate work you have done to achieve a particular nursing competency. However, keep in mind that you must maintain confidentiality at all times. If you plan to use pictures or videos you will need written consent before including them.

Summary

Portfolios are becoming the norm and all students and nurses should develop a portfolio whether or not it is mandatory. There are different types of portfolios, such as academic portfolios, which demonstrate learning and competency, and professional portfolios, which demonstrate development and competency in specific areas. Portfolios may be developed in hard copy or in an electronic format. Although the electronic format is preferred it is not mandatory. The key to portfolio development is to follow an organized framework and be sure all the documents are of highest quality. There is a plethora of information that one can include in an individual portfolio. However, it is important to follow the caveat that quality trumps quantity.

Discussion Questions

1. What is the purpose of a portfolio?
2. Discuss the key components of an academic portfolio.
3. Discuss the key components of a professional portfolio.
4. What are some issues identified with academic portfolios?
5. Realizing that all portfolios differ, what are some of the common items and documentation that should be included in a professional portfolio (According to Casey and Egan [2010])?
6. What are the four steps that Oermann (2002) outlines for professional portfolio development?
7. Which countries require registered nurses to develop portfolios?
8. What is a "Best Work" portfolio?
9. What is a "Growth and Development" portfolio?
10. Who should you ask to review your portfolio?

SUGGESTED LEARNING ACTIVITIES

- Develop a portfolio using one of the templates included in the chapter.
- Explore online portfolio development programs.
- Interview a nursing professor or staff nurse who has developed a portfolio.

REFERENCES

Byrne, M., Delarose, T., King, C., Leske, J., Sapnas, K., & Schroeter, K. (2007). Continued professional competence and portfolios. *Journal of Trauma Nursing, 14*(1), 24–31.

Casey, D., & Egan, D. (2010). The use of professional portfolios and profiles for career enhancement. *British Journal of Community Nursing, 15*(11), 547–552.

Davis, M., Ponnamperuma, G., & Ker, J. (2009). Student perceptions of a portfolio assessment process. *Medical Education, 43*(1), 89–98. doi:10.1111/j.1365-2923.2008.03250.x

Driessen, E., Muijtjens, A., van Tartwijk, J., & van der Vleuten, C. P. (2007). Web- or paper-based portfolios: Is there a difference? *Medical Education, 41*(11), 1067–1073.

Green, J., Wyllie, A., & Jackson, D. (2014). Electronic portfolios in nursing education: A review of the literature. *Nurse Education in Practice, 14*(1), 4–8. doi:10.1016/j.nepr.2013.08.011

Hawks, S. J. (2012). The use of electronic portfolios in nurse anesthesia education and practice. *AANA Journal, 80*(2), 89–93.

Joyce, P. (2005). A framework for portfolio development in postgraduate nursing practice. *Journal of Clinical Nursing, 14*(4), 456–463. doi:10.1111/j.1365-2702.2004.01075.x

McMullan, M., Endacott, R., Gray, M., Jasper, M., Miller, C., Scholes, J., & Webb, C. (2003). Portfolios and assessment of competence: A review of the literature. *Journal of Advanced Nursing, 41*(3), 283–294. doi:10.1046/j.1365-2648.2003.02528.x

Meister, L., Heath, J., Andrews, J., & Tingen, M. (2002). Professional nursing portfolios: A global perspective. *MEDSURG Nursing, 11*(4), 177–182.

Nairn, S., O'Brien, E., Traynor, V., Williams, G., Chapple, M., & Johnson, S. (2006). Student nurses' knowledge, skills and attitudes towards the use of portfolios in a school of nursing. *Journal of Clinical Nursing, 15*(12), 1509–1520. doi:10.1111/j.1365-2702.2005.01432.x

Oermann, M. (2002). Developing a professional portfolio in nursing. *Orthopaedic Nursing, 21*(2), 73–78.

Rossetti, J., Oldenburg, N., Robertson, J., Coyer, S. M., Koren, M. E., Peters, B., & Musker, K. (2012). Creating a culture of evidence in nursing education using student portfolios. *International Journal of Nursing Education Scholarship, 9*(1), 1–14.

Sinclair, P. M., Bowen, L., & Donkin, B. (2013). Professional nephrology nursing portfolios: Maintaining competence to practise. *Renal Society of Australasia Journal, 9*(1), 35+. Retrieved from http://go.galegroup.com.libezcnr.idm.oclc.org/ps/i.do?id=GALE%7CA341368797&v=2.1&u=nysl_me_gilllib&it=r&p=PPNU&sw=w&asid=655cfb6b5164bc641836069d231f13b4

Thompson, T. (2011). Electronic portfolios for professional advancement. *Clinical Nurse Specialist: The Journal for Advanced Nursing Practice, 25*(4), 169–170. doi:10.1097/NUR.0b013e318222a680

Timmins, F., & Dunne, P. (2009). An exploration of the current use and benefit of nursing student portfolios. *Nurse Education Today, 29*(3), 330–341. doi:10.1016/j.nedt.2008.12.010

Williams, G., Park, J., Traynor, V., Nairn, S., O'Brien, E., Chapple, M., & Johnson, S. (2009). Lecturers' and students' perceptions of portfolios in an English school of nursing. *Journal of Clinical Nursing, 18*(8), 1113–1122. doi:10.1111/j.1365-2702.2008.02553.x

CHAPTER 5

Quality and Safety Issues

The very first requirement in a hospital is that it should do the sick no harm.

—Florence Nightingale

OBJECTIVES

After reading this chapter the reader will be able to:

- Discuss the JCAHO (Joint Commission on Accreditation of Healthcare Organizations) national safety goals
- Discuss issues related to patient safety
- Discuss issues related to quality of care
- Understand the Quality and Safety Education for Nurses (QSEN) competencies
- Describe the knowledge, skills, and attitudes of each QSEN competency

Quality and safety are two concepts that must be ingrained in every health care professional's very being and incorporated into daily practice. Every single day we read about issues regarding negative patient outcomes and poor quality of care. These issues run the gamut from falls and medication errors to poor quality of care and wrong site/side surgery. It is vital that all health care professionals understand the significance of quality and safety, ways to improve patient outcomes, and prevent adverse events. We must all do our part individually and collectively to promote and maintain a culture of safety. Although health care professionals strive to provide high quality of care, the landmark report by the Institute of Medicine *To Err Is Human: Building a Safer Health System* highlighted the pervasive nature of medical errors and poor quality of care in various health care organizations (Kohn, Corrigan, & Donaldson, 1999, as cited in Hunt, 2012). According to the report, which was published in 1999, "the estimated cost of medical errors was between $17 billion and $29 billion at hospitals across the country, with death rates between 44,000 and 98,000" (Hunt, 2012, para. 1). When this report was initially published the nation was shocked and dismayed. How did this happen? Why were there so many errors? And why were we unaware of this alarming situation? When reading this one might think there was something sinister occurring throughout the health care industry. In reality it wasn't that hospitals were covering up the errors, although they did not publicize them. When an error occurred an internal investigation was done and the findings would be reported to the appropriate regulatory agency. However, there was not a national database that was shared with the general public or with other health care organizations so no one was aware of the staggering number of adverse events that were occurring in every organization around the country. The 1999 report prompted a swift response from the health care industry and regulatory agencies, such as The Joint Commission and the Agency for Healthcare Research and Quality. Both of these agencies developed standards for health care agencies to follow such as "voluntary nationwide reporting" and the "Just Culture Initiative" (Hunt, 2012, para. 2). These initiatives will be more thoroughly discussed in another section of this chapter. Although we have made significant strides in patient safety and quality of care we still have far too many errors and experts continue to investigate this issue and develop strategies for promoting a culture of quality and safety. An example of this is the Robert Wood Johnson Foundation and its funding and support of Quality and Safety Education for Nurses (QSEN) competencies. The QSEN competencies were developed in response to high error rates with the premise being that student nurses achieve these competencies as students and will then be able to provide safe and effective high-quality care and serve as role models to other nurses (QSEN, 2014).

This chapter focuses on various aspects of patient safety and quality. An overview of patient safety and quality issues will be provided in addition to the measures that have been taken by health care organizations in response to the Institute of Medicine's report and the requirements of regulatory agencies, such as The Joint Commission (TJC), and the Centers for Medicare & Medicaid Services (CMS), and the Department of Health (DOH). The QSEN competencies will be thoroughly discussed especially in relation to your role as a student and novice nurse.

SAFETY AND QUALITY

"Safety" and "quality" are two umbrella terms for a multitude of patient issues and initiatives. Although they are related they are not the same, thus it is crucial to possess a foundational understanding of these concepts, especially in regard to the role you play in providing safe and effective quality of care. Furthermore, these are also foundational to achieving the QSEN competencies.

Safety is a familiar term and something we learned about as little children. For example, we learn about fire safety, safe environments, car safety, and pedestrian safety, just to name a few. Patient safety is what we focus on in the health care setting and there are all types of regulations that we all must follow. For example, The Joint Commission is an accrediting agency that has focused on safety and quality for the past 60 years (TJC, 2013). According to their website TJC, formally known as JCAHO, is an agency that accredits and certifies over 20,000 health care agencies throughout the United States (TJC, 2013a). Since its inception, The Joint Commission has developed and implemented a multitude of quality and safety issues in an effort to improve safety and quality within the health care setting. The Joint Commission revises and updates its standards based on current practice guidelines, quality and safety issues, and current evidence and research. Earning accreditation is technically not mandatory, although it would be difficult for a health care agency to be successful without TJC's seal of approval (TJC, 2013a). Organizations are usually surveyed every 3 years and must demonstrate their compliance with each standard required by TJC. As a student and a new nurse you will need to understand the role that The Joint Commission plays in your organization. Your academic institution is also subject to accreditation but the agencies and standards used are different. When The Joint Commission comes to survey an organization everyone must be prepared and knowledgeable about the standards. This includes students and volunteers. When you go to clinical sites as a student you will either attend classes or complete self-learning modules on mandatory topics such as fire safety, standard precautions, and patient safety. These are not just "busy work" they contain vital information that will help you maintain a safe environment for all. The Joint Commission has implemented a myriad of standards to promote positive patient outcomes. Many of these were in response to the 1990 report. For example:

- "Do-not-use list" of abbreviations
- Advancing effective communication, cultural competence, and patient- and family-centered care

- National Patient Safety Goals (NPSG)
- Infection control
- Sentinel event alert

Health care organizations develop policies and procedures that guide staff in the provision of care. The policies also are developed in accordance with The Joint Commission and other regulatory agencies such as the CMS and DOH.

Although quality and safety have always been at the forefront of all health care organizations, regulatory, and accrediting agencies after the 1999 *To Err Is Human* report revealed that our organizations were fraught with quality and safety issues; there was a major shift and new standards were developed at a rapid rate. For example, in 2001 The Joint Commission issued an alert on medical abbreviations. These abbreviations had been used for years but on investigation were related to multiple medication errors. For example, the abbreviation "U" for units, used when ordering insulin, was extremely dangerous. Because of unclear handwriting and lack of knowledge 10 units of insulin could be mistaken for 100 units of insulin. This high dose can lead to hypoglycemia, coma, and even death. Therefore, the entire word "units" must be completely spelled out for any drug that is ordered in units. Because of misinterpretations of medications it is no longer acceptable to abbreviate names of medications. There are several other dangerous abbreviations that must be avoided and you can find additional information about the "Do Not Use" list on their website (TJC, 2013b).

The National Patient Safety Goals are yet another safety initiative of The Joint Commission that were developed in an effort to mitigate patients' risks inherent in the health care arena. They were originally developed in 2002 by a panel of interprofessional health care experts and went into effect in 2003 (TJC, 2013c). For example:

- Using two patient identifiers, such as name and medical record number
- Developing a list of acceptable and unacceptable abbreviations
- Removing potassium and high concentrated sodium chloride from patient units
- Preventing wrong-site and wrong-patient surgery

Since the inception of the NPSGs, The Joint Commission has continued to develop them further and new goals have been implemented. For example, in 2008 goals were added regarding patient falls, surgical fires, involving patients in their care, and improving recognition and response to changes in patients' conditions (Catalano & Fickensher, 2008).

Reducing pressure ulcers is also included in the goals and in 2014 a new goal on safe clinical alarm management in hospitals and critical access hospitals will be introduced in two phases. Phase 1 began on January 1, 2014, and requires hospitals to establish alarm safety as an organizational goal and identify the most vital alarms in their institution. Phase 2 will be implemented in January 2016 and will require hospitals to develop policies and procedures and educate staff on this safety goal (TJC, 2014). The Sentinel Event Policy was instituted in 1996 by The Joint Commission (TJC, 2013d) and is described as an "unexpected occurrence involving death or serious physical or psychological injury, or the risk thereof. Serious injuries specifically include a loss of limb or function" (TJC, 2009, para. 1).

When a sentinel event (unexpected death, suicide, rape, surgery on wrong individual or body part, infant abduction) occurs, hospitals are required to conduct a "root cause analysis" to determine the cause of the adverse event. Although hospitals are not required to notify The Joint Commission it is advisable to inform them. As a student or a nurse you would not be expected to report such an event. However, if you were involved in the event you must complete an incident/occurrence report and notify your clinical instructor if you are a student, or your supervisor if working. Most likely you will be interviewed as part of the investigation as to the cause of the adverse event. Although it is frightening to make an error it is vital to report it immediately so as to protect the patients and your license. Many hospitals view adverse events as a systems issue and thoroughly evaluate the cause and events of each occurrence. The best way to prevent errors is to follow your hospital's policies and procedures and seek guidance when required. Effective July 2013, The Joint Commission expanded their sentinel event policy to include injury to health care workers. The reasoning behind this is that they expect all organizations to promote safety for patients, families, and employees (Hospital Employee Health, 2013).

Infection control is another issue that has been at the forefront of regulatory agencies, administration, and all health care employees. Florence Nightingale is credited with identifying hand washing and cleanliness as a significant factor in patient mortality. Hand hygiene is so simple and easy to comply with, however it is a well-known fact that many health care workers and the general public do not wash their hands as often as they should. Hospital acquired infections are a significant threat to patients (Creedon, 2005). Aston (2013) posits that due to the growing threat of antibiotic-resistant bacteria strains and new Medicare penalties for hospitals with the most infections there has been a concerted effort by government and hospitals to ramp up their infection control programs.

Every day hospitals strive to prevent infections and protect patients, families, and employees. Unfortunately, in light of current issues with resistant pathogens this is an extremely daunting task. This is complicated by the fact that despite the development of evidenced-based practice guidelines on hand hygiene, compliance rates remain alarmingly low (Creedon, 2005). The Joint Commission, the Department of Health, the Centers for Medicare & Medicaid Services, the Centers for Disease Control, the World Health Organization, along with other agencies have very strict standards relating to infection control. Hospitals must provide yearly infection control courses and in New York all licensed health care workers must complete a state-approved infection control course every 4 years. Universal precautions are employed by all health care workers when there is potential exposure to a patient's blood or bodily fluid, which means every patient is considered to be potentially infected with blood-borne pathogens such as HIV and hepatitis. Health care workers are required to wear gloves when the potential of coming in contact with a patient's blood or bodily fluids exists. Personal protective equipment (PPE), such as gowns, gloves, masks, booties, and head coverings, should also be considered if the situation warrants this level of protection. Some patients will need to be in isolation due to the nature of their disease and when this occurs you will be provided with clear guidelines as to the use of PPE. However, it is always in your purview to include additional PPE if you feel the situation necessitates it. For example, you may need to wear a waterproof gown or goggles if a patient is experiencing projectile vomiting, or "bleeding out." Remember that hand washing remains the single most effective way to prevent the spread of infections. Hand hygiene should be done before and after each patient contact and before and after removing gloves and whenever hands become potentially contaminated. It is important to follow your organization's policies and procedures. "According to estimates from the Centers for Disease Control and Prevention (CDC), each year nearly two million patients in the United States get an infection in hospitals, and about 90,000 of these patients die as a result of their infection" (CDC, 2004, as cited in TJC, 2014a). The key to addressing this issue is to use best practices and implement strategies that are aimed at changing the behavior of health care workers so that they are in full compliance with these practices (Aston, 2013). Because of changes in the CMS policies, hospitals are no longer being reimbursed for hospital-acquired pressure ulcers and infections such as urinary tract infections. Although progress has been slow in reducing hospital-acquired infections there is some promising news: Central-line associated bloodstream infections (CLABSIs) "fell 41% in 2011" (Aston, 2011, p. 51). Clearly we have much work to do but we are certainly moving in the right direction. You can do your part by adhering to strict guidelines and advocating for your patients by reminding others about the importance of infection control. Another key initiative of The Joint Commission relates to communication and cultural diversity. According to the Joint Commission (2010):

> A hospital must embed effective communication, cultural competence, and patient- and family-centered care practices into the core activities of its system of care delivery—not considering them stand-alone initiatives—to truly meet the needs of the patients, families, and communities served. (p. 4)

The Joint Commission (2010) published *Advancing Effective Communication, Cultural Competence, and Patient- and Family-Centered Care: A Roadmap for Hospitals* to serve as a guide to health care organizations as they strive to meet these standards. The Joint Commission has many standards that relate to virtually every aspect of health care organizations and all health care employees must be knowledgeable about these standards and how they affect practice. The Joint Commission website contains a wealth of information so it is highly advisable for you to explore this site.

There are so many other agencies and websites you can explore to further your knowledge on these vital issues. Certainly as a student you will be introduced to many of these issues and you will continue to learn about these ever-changing initiatives throughout your entire journey. As a student and later as a registered nurse you should always engage in self-directed learning and approach each day with a spirit of inquiry.

JUST CULTURE

The health care arena is fraught with errors and despite our best efforts to prevent them there are a myriad of factors that may lead to an adverse event. Due in part to the two landmark reports such as *To Err Is Human: Building a Safer Health System,* and the follow-up report *Keeping Patients Safe: Transforming the Work Environment of Nurses* there has been a shift from "blame and shame" to a "just culture" initiative (Kohn et al., 1999; Committee on the Work Environment for Nurses and Patient Safety, 2004; as cited in Hunt, 2012). To develop a comprehensive safety program we must first understand the significance and causes of the myriad adverse effects that occur almost daily throughout health care organizations. Applying the principles of the nursing process can guide us in the continued development of safety programs. However, in the past many individuals and organizations were hesitant to openly share their vulnerability. Shifting the focus to a more systems-wide issue promotes openness and sharing of problems for the greater good. It is important to note that this philosophical shift does not protect individuals who are guilty of gross misconduct that results in harm toward patients (Miranda & Olexa, 2013). "A just culture focuses on identifying and addressing systems issues that lead individuals to engage in unsafe behaviors, while maintaining individual accountability by establishing zero tolerance for reckless behavior" (Agency for Healthcare Research and Quality, 2012, para. 5). Miranda and Olexa (2013) share some very important points regarding our current approach to safety, citing the need for less government regulation and more personal accountability and more input from nursing leaders. Although others agree, experts such as Patricia Stone point out that infection control is not just a nursing responsibility and we need to approach this from an interdisciplinary perspective (Wilson Pecci, 2014). We are all accountable for our own actions and must be sure to be guided by our Nurse Practice Act while providing high-quality safe and effective nursing care.

QUALITY OF CARE

Health care organizations continually seek to provide and improve quality care for their patients. Most hospitals have quality improvement departments and personnel who focus on data collection, analysis, and benchmarking of patient outcomes data. "With growing concern about hospital care quality and attention to the need for improvement of care, quality improvement (QI) has become an administrative mandate in US hospitals" (Izumi, 2012, p. 260). Izumi posits "There are three interrelated but slightly different views about the cause of the health care quality problem" (p. 261). The three factors relate to inefficient health care systems, staffing shortages, and inadequate quality improvement initiatives (Izumi, 2012). Therefore health care organizations measure many different quality issues; some relate to the national database, such as pressure ulcers, and others relate to issues that are specific to an organization, such as blood transfusion. Certainly safety is related to quality and is an important area to be benchmarked. However, quality-improvement programs also measure compliance to national and/or hospital policies. Staffing levels are also related to patient safety and quality. Aiken et al. (2002) conducted a cross-sectional analysis of 10,184 nurses and found a relationship between nurse workload and patient mortality. There is a 7% increase in mortality rates when nurses have more than four postop patients to care for. However, decisions to alter staffing should be based on empirical evidence. A successful quality-improvement program requires input from all the employees because each employee plays a role in patient safety and quality of care.

The Joint Commission has specific standards relating to quality improvement and patient outcomes. The National Database of Nurse Quality Indicators was developed in 1998 (Montalvo, 2007). "Evaluating the quality of nursing practice began when Florence Nightingale identified nursing's role in health care quality and began to measure patient outcomes" (Montalvo, 2007, para. 2). Nursing- sensitive indicators include pressure ulcers, patient falls, vascular catheter-associated infections, and catheter-related urinary tract infections (Nance, 2008). Although these are identified as nursing-sensitive indicators one must realize that it is often hard to isolate one caregiver in relation to quality and safety. For example, a patient may fall while in the care of the physician or physical therapist. Therefore, it is important to collaborate with all members of the health care team. Documentation is key to demonstrating adherence to policies and procedures and provision of care. Oftentimes nurses and other health care providers have provided the expected level of care but fail to document it. There is an old saying, "If it wasn't documented it wasn't done." The legalities of documentation along with other legal issues will most likely be included in your curriculum and during your orientation you will be introduced to the documentation system of your health care organization. You will also learn about quality improvement and nursing sensitive indicators. However, it behooves you to be a self-directed learner and learn as much as you can about this and other issues relating to your practice.

QUALITY AND SAFETY EDUCATION FOR NURSES

The Robert Wood Johnson Foundation has been and continues to be a strong supporter of nursing and health care with a focus on improving patient outcomes. "In 2005, the Robert Wood Johnson Foundation (RWJF) funded a national study to evaluate and enhance undergraduate and graduate nursing students about patient safety and quality because nursing plays a central role in patient outcomes" (Hunt 2012, para. 4). The result of this undertaking was the development and implementation of the QSEN initiative. In 2005 a panel of experts was selected by RWJF to develop a program that would be included in all undergraduate nursing curriculums; the premise being that it was vital for future nurses to develop the knowledge, skills, and attitudes required to promote quality of care and maintain safety in all health care organizations. This cadre of new clinicians would then serve as role models in their respective health care organizations (QSEN, 2014). This project initially had three phases and funding was provided to the American Association of Colleges of Nurses (AACN) and The University of North

Carolina by the Robert Wood Johnson Foundation to support its development and implementation (QSEN, 2014).

The QSEN project included four phases. Phase I was devoted to developing the QSEN competencies and a plan for dissemination among schools of nursing. The expert panel developed six competencies (detailed in the next section), which included five competencies from the Institute of Medicine (QSEN, 2014). In addition to these definitions, sets of knowledge, skills, and attitudes for each of the six competencies were created for use in nursing prelicensure programs (Cronenwett et al., 2007, as cited in QSEN, 2014). Phase II (2007–2009) focused on development of the QSEN website to share information, strategies and resources, and the integration of the competencies in selected pilot schools. In Phase III (2009–2012) faculty workshops were sponsored by RWJF and held by the AACN to develop a cadre of faculty who were well versed in the QSEN curriculum. Faculty who completed the QSEN training were then expected to participate in "train the trainers" at their academic institutions. Phase IV (2012–present) is focused on graduate faculty and students (QSEN, 2014). Many health care organizations are also beginning to include QSEN in their staff development and competency programs.

QSEN COMPETENCIES

There are six QSEN competencies and each one is defined and includes competency statements relating to the knowledge, skills, and attitudes that reflect achievement of the various competencies. The six competencies are patient-centered care, teamwork and collaboration, evidence-based practice (EBP), quality improvement (QI), safety, and informatics (Hunt, 2012; QSEN, 2014).

The first competency, patient-centered care, places the patient at the center of care and serves as a reminder to us all that we must always include the patient's personal expectations in our plan of care. The definition of patient-centered care according to the expert panel is "recognize the patient or designee as the source of control and full partner in providing compassionate and coordinated care based on respect for the patient's preferences, values, and needs" (Cronenwett et al., 2007, p. 123). Demonstrating competency in knowledge, skills, and attitudes would be evident in the student's understanding of the unique holistic needs of patients, providing patient-centered care, and valuing the patient's wishes.

The second competency is teamwork and collaboration, which is defined as the ability to "function effectively within nursing and inter-professional teams, fostering open communication, mutual respect, and shared decision-making to achieve quality patient care" (Cronenwett et al., 2007, p. 124). Demonstrating competency in knowledge, skills, and attitudes would be evident in the student's understanding of the scope and practice of various members of the interdisciplinary team, assuming the role of team member, and valuing teamwork (Cronenwett et al., 2007).

Evidenced-based practice is the third competency and is defined as the ability to "integrate best current evidence with clinical expertise and patient/family preferences and values for delivery of optimal health care (Cronenwett et al., 2007, p. 125). Achievement of the knowledge, skills, and attitudes required for this competency include the ability to describe evidenced-based practice, use evidenced-based practice, and value the importance of reading current research (Cronenwett et al., 2007).

The next competency is quality improvement, which is defined as the ability to "use data to monitor the outcomes of care processes and use improvement methods to design and test changes to continuously improve the quality and safety of health care systems" (Cronenwett et al., 2007, p. 126). Demonstrating competency in knowledge, skills, and attitudes would be evident in a student's understanding of the quality-improvement process, participate in a root cause analysis, and value the use of measurement in patient care (Cronenwett et al., 2007).

Safety is the fifth competency and is defined as "Minimize risk of harm to patients and providers through both system effectiveness and individual performance" (Cronenwett et al., 2007, p. 128). Achievement of knowledge, skills, and attitudes includes the ability to discuss the impact of national safety programs, use strategies to reduce harm to patients, and value one's role in preventing errors (Cronenwett et al., 2007).

The last competency is informatics, which is defined as the ability to "use information and technology to communicate, manage knowledge, mitigate error, and support decision-making" (Cronenwett et al., 2007, p. 129). Demonstrating competency in knowledge, skills, and attitudes would be evident in the student's ability to explain why skills in information technology relate to safe patient care, the ability to use the electronic health record, and value nurses' involvement in the design of information technologies that support patient care (Cronenwett et al., 2007).

There are many other competency statements for each QSEN competency and these have been further delineated into stages so that students can progress from novice, beginner, to advanced. You should first be introduced to the QSEN competencies in your foundational nursing course, where the focus is more on knowledge development. Following this the QSEN competencies should be integrated and threaded in to all of your nursing courses throughout the curriculum. You should also be a self-directed learner and explore the QSEN website for additional information. There are also modules available on the American Association of Colleges of Nurses website. QSEN is extremely important and your future places of employment will expect you to have achieved these competencies as a student and continue to expand on them throughout your nursing career. Furthermore, many recruiters will assess your knowledge of QSEN upon interview so you want to be sure to be well prepared.

SUMMARY

This chapter focused on patient safety, quality of care, and the QSEN competencies. The significance of these factors in regard to both the student and nursing role was discussed. All nurses and health care workers play a significant role in the delivery of high quality of care and the promotion of positive patient outcomes that are based on current research and evidence.

DISCUSSION QUESTIONS

1. Describe the role of The Joint Commission in health care.
2. Select three of the National Patient Safety Goals from inception to current-day practice. Have they had a positive impact on patient safety?
3. What additional goals should be added to the current list of the National Patient Safety Goals?
4. What other agencies inform safety and quality in the health care setting?

5. Discuss quality of care in the health care setting.
6. What are *nursing sensitive indicators*? Do you agree with this list?
7. Discuss the history and phases of QSEN. Do you believe that QSEN has improved quality and safety in the health care setting?
8. List and describe the six QSEN competencies.
9. Describe the purpose of quality improvement.
10. What are the key components of the "just culture" initiative?

SUGGESTED LEARNING ACTIVITIES

- Develop a quality improvement project.
- Read the report *To Err Is Human* and reflect on its contribution to health care.
- Read *Advancing Effective Communication, Cultural Competence, and Patient-and Family-Centered Care: A Roadmap for Hospitals.*
- Write an essay on the impact of The Joint Commission's National Patient Safety Goals.
- Interview a nursing leader about safety and quality initiatives in their organization.
- Develop a project related to QSEN.
- Write a reflective journal on how the QSEN competencies informed your practice.

REFERENCES

Agency for Healthcare Research and Quality. (n.d.). *Safety culture*. Retrieved from http://www.ahrq.gov.

Agency for Healthcare Research and Quality (AHRQ). (2012). *Patient safety primers, safety culture*. Retrieved from http://psnet.ahrq.gov/primer.aspx?primerID

Aiken, L. H., Clarke, S. P., Sloane, D. M., Sochalski, J., & Silber, J. H. (2002). Hospital nurse staffing and patient mortality, nurse burnout, and job dissatisfaction. *Journal of the American Medical Association, 288*(16), 1987–1999.

Aston, G. (2013). Infection prevention: Hospitals step it up. *H&HN: Hospitals & Health Networks, 87*(11), 50–53.

Catalano, K., & Fickenscher, K. (2008). Complying with the 2008 National Patient Safety Goals. *AORN Journal, 87*(3), 547–556. doi:10.1016/j.aorn.2007.12.029

Centers for Disease Control and Prevention. (2004). *National nosocomial infections surveillance system.* Retrieved from http://www.cdc.gov/nhsn/PDFs/dataStat/NNIS_2004.pdf

Committee on the Work Environment for Nurses and Patient Safety. (2003). *Keeping patients safe: Transforming the work environment of nurses.* Washington, DC: National Academies Press. Retrieved from http://www.iom.edu/Reports/2003/Keeping-Patients-Safe-Transforming-the-Work-Environment-of-Nurses.aspx

Creedon, S. (2005). Health care workers' hand decontamination practices: Compliance with recommended guidelines. *Journal of Advanced Nursing, 51*(3), 208–216. doi:10.1111/j.1365-2648.2005.03490.x

Cronenwett, L., Sherwood, G., Barnsteiner, J., Disch, J., Johnson, J., Mitchell, P.,... Warren, J., (2007). Quality and safety education for nurses. *Nursing Outlook, 55*(3), 122–131.

Hunt, D. (2012). QSEN Competencies: A bridge to practice. *Nursing Made Incredibly Easy, 10*(5), 1–3. Retrieved from http://journals.lww.com/nursingmadeincrediblyeasy/Fulltext/2012/09000/QSEN_competencies__A_bridge_to_practice.1.aspx

Izumi, S. (2012). Quality improvement in nursing: Administrative mandate or Professional responsibility? *Nursing Forum, 47*(4), 260–267. doi:10.1111/j.1744-6198.2012.00283.x

The Joint Commission. (2009). Facts about the Joint Commission policies. Accessed at http://www.jointcommission.org/Sentinel_Event_Policy_and_Procedures

The Joint Commission. (2010). *Advancing effective communication, cultural competence, and patient- and family-centered care: Roadmap for hospitals.* Oakbrook Terrace, IL: Author.

The Joint Commission. (2013). *The Joint Commission history.* Accessed at http://www.jointcommission.org.

The Joint Commission. (2013a). *Certification handbook.* Retrieved from http://www.jointcommission.org/assets/1/18/2013_HCSS_Certification_Guide.pdf

The Joint Commission. (2013b). *Facts about the official "do not use" list.* Accessed at https://www.jointcommission.org/assets/1/18/Do_Not_Use_List.pdf

The Joint Commission. (2013c). *Facts about the National Patient Safety Goals.* Accessed at https://www.jointcommission.org.

The Joint Commission. (2013d). Serious HCW injuries are now sentinel events. *Hospital Employee Health, 32*(2), 13–15.

The Joint Commission. (2014). *2014 National Patient Safety Goals.* Accessed at https://www.jointcommission.org.

The Joint Commission. (2014a). *Sentinel event alert: Infection control related sentinel events.* Retrieved from http://www.jointcommission.org/sentinel_event_alert_issue_28_infection_control_related_sentinel_events/

Joint Commission on Accreditation of Healthcare Organizations. (2003). 2003 JCAHO National Patient Safety Goals. *Kansas Nurse*, 78(6), 7-8.

Kohn , L., Corrigan, J., & Donaldson, M.; Institute of Medicine. (1999). *To err is human: Building a safer health system.* Washington, DC: National Academies Press.

Miranda, J., & Olexa, G. A. (2013). Creating a just culture. *Pennsylvania Nurse*, 68(4), 4–10.

Montalvo, I. (2007). The National Database of Nursing Quality Indicators (NDNQI). *Online Journal of Issues in Nursing*, 12(3).

Nance, B. (2008). Nurse sensitive indicators: a staff nurse perspective. *Oklahoma Nurse*, 53(4), 7.

Pauly-O'Neill, S., Prion, S., & Nguyen, H. (2013). Comparison of quality and safety education for nurses (QSEN)-related student experiences during pediatric clinical and simulation rotations. *Journal of Nursing Education*, 52(9), 534–538. doi:10.3928

Prepare for enhanced scrutiny on infection control as regulators clamp down on unsafe practices related to health care-associated infections. (2013). *ED Management*, 25(12), 1–3.

QSEN: Quality and Safety Education for Nurses. (2014). Retrieved from http://qsen.org/

Wilson Pecci, A. (2014). HAIs: Not just a nursing problem. HealthLeaders Media. Accessed at https://www.healthleadersmedia.com.

CHAPTER 6

Legal, Moral, and Ethical Issues

In just about every area of society, there's nothing more important than ethics.

—Henry Paulson

OBJECTIVES

After reading this chapter the reader will be able to:

- Understand the legal, moral, and ethical issues that inform his or her practice
- Discuss the legalities of professional practice
- Describe malpractice and negligence
- Understand the ethical principles
- Describe the legal, moral, and ethical issues in health care and nursing practice

The nature of nursing and health care is one that is filled with a myriad of legal, moral, and ethical issues and one must understand these issues and how they inform professional practice. One must also be guided by legal, moral, and ethical concepts when providing health care. You may refer to Chapter 1 for more detailed information about the Nurse Practice Act and ANA (American Nurses Association) Code of Ethics. Legal issues relate to provision of patient care, the Nurse Practice Act, adhering to policies and procedures, and proper documentation. Moral issues focus on doing what is right and not just whether or not it is legally required. Ethical issues include matters such as do-not-resuscitate orders and the provision or withholding of care. Ethical issues usually have no right or wrong solution but are certainly intertwined with legal and moral factors. As a student and eventually a nurse you will be faced with many legal, moral, and ethical decisions. Some of these issues will be addressed individually, whereas others will require a team approach. Examples of different types of individual and organizational situations will be discussed throughout the chapter.

ETHICAL ISSUES IN NURSING AND HEALTH CARE

"Ethics" is the field of study that addresses issues of what is morally acceptable and how this informs behavior. Many professions are guided by a code of ethics specific to their practice. Nursing ethics deal specifically with moral and ethical issues that nurses face in their working environments. These situations require thoughtful inquiry and analysis of beliefs, values, and attitudes toward a particular ethical issue (Harding, 2013). Arries (2014) posits that nurses need to find a balance between quality and safety, which he refers to as "ethics quality in nursing" (p. 4). Patient safety and the ethical imperative are closely intertwined and for all intents and purposes cannot be viewed as separate entities. "When seeking moral arguments for patient safety, the ethical imperative can be seen as driven from the original mission and the aim of health care systems" (Kangasniemi, Vaismoradi, Jasper, & Turunen, 2013, p. 905). As health care providers we are charged with the moral, legal, and ethical responsibility to promote human dignity and positive patient outcomes using resources in a manner that decreases the financial burden of health care on our society. Although ethical care is not mandated it is inherent in one's professional code of conduct and if one is derelict in his or her duties may be subject to legal and moral consequences (Kangasniemi et al. 2013). Health care organizations have ethical committees that are comprised of various experts. It is important to have at least a basic knowledge of the ethical issues and the ethical principles that guide decision making when you encounter and ethical issues. Certainly in nursing school ethics will be taught either in an individual course or threaded within the curriculum. However, ethical issues are complex and you will need to continue to learn about the various ethical issues that you may face throughout your nursing career. There are different theories and principles that guide experts when they are analyzing an ethical dilemma and most organizations will convene their ethics committee when dealing with complex issues. Some examples of ethical dilemmas are:

- The use of artificial nutrition and hydration
- Advance directives and do-not-resuscitate orders (DNRs)

- End-of-life care
- Abortions
- Patients who are in a persistent vegetative state

These issues are complex and many people have conflicting views on what is best for the patient. For example, the family may "want everything done," whereas the health care practitioners may "want to avoid causing the patient further discomfort." It is important to note that there are no right or wrong decisions when it comes to an ethical issue. To help guide the process, theories and principles of ethics are used by individuals who are considered experts and who comprise the ethics panel. There are several theories that may be used by the panel. For example, utilitarianism, deontology, and virtue ethics are just a few of the theories that inform ethical decision making. "Utilitarianism is the moral theory that holds that an action is judged as good or bad in relation to the consequence, outcome, or end result that is derived from it" (Burkhart & Nathanial, 2002, p. 28) and considers the good of the whole rather than the individual. Virtue ethics relates to "right and wrong" and concepts such as compassion and truthfulness. Deontology is based on what the philosopher Kant describes as the "rightness or wrongness" of a situation and that decisions should be made on the basis of truth and respect (Burkhart & Nathaniel, 2002).

Ethical committees also use various ethical principles to guide them throughout the process of ethical decision making. The five main principles are:

- Beneficence
- Nonmaleficence
- Autonomy and informed consent
- Truthfulness and confidentiality
- Justice

The principle of beneficence relates to the moral obligation of performing acts for the benefit of others. We need to "do good" and consider our actions at all times. Most health care providers would never intentionally harm a patient; however, failing to follow policy and procedures is a failure to fulfill one's obligations. Moral obligations include preventing harm, protecting others, helping persons with disabilities, and rescuing patients in danger (Beauchamp & Childress, 2001). For example, nurses evaluate medication orders to be sure they are not harmful to the patient. If they are concerned with a particular medication order they question the health care provider and consult with their administrators to ensure patient safety. Admittedly it can be difficult to question a health care practitioner, especially as a student or new nurse. However, one must always be guided by moral, ethical, and legal principles. The ethical principle of nonmaleficence requires one to protect the patient from harm (Burkhart & Nathaniel, 2013). Learning the safety goals, becoming a lifelong learner, following proper protocols, and using research and current evidence are all ways of preventing harm to patients. All patients and/or their families or health care agents have the right to autonomy and to decide the type of health care they desire. Beauchamp and Childress (2001) posit, "Virtually all theories of autonomy agree that two conditions are essential for autonomy: (1) liberty (independence from controlling influences) and (2) agency (capacity for intentional action)" (p. 58). It is vital to serve as a patient/family advocate and ensure that patient rights are protected. "Informed consent provides legal protection of a patient's right to personal autonomy" (Burkhardt & Nathaniel, 2002, p. 209). The patient or patient's surrogate is given the opportunity to make an autonomous choice regarding consent to procedures, treatments, and refusal of such procedures. Informed consent is a legal and ethical process that involves the giving of information by the health care provider. The information must be comprehensive and include the risks, benefits, and alternatives to the procedure. The following standards are used in determining adequacy of information: (a) the professional practice standard, (b) the reasonable person standard, (c) the subjective standard. Patients should be given the opportunity to seek clarification and efforts should be made to verify that the information was understood. Consent is the ability to assess or reject the recommended procedure. The person should not be coerced into making the decision. The nurse's role in this process is to witness and authenticate the signature as well as verify the competency of the patient and his/her understanding of the procedure, including risks, benefits, and alternatives (Burkhardt & Nathaniel, 2002). For example, a patient should be given the opportunity to make informed end-of-life care decisions while she or he is still healthy and possesses the cognitive ability to make decisions. As a nurse you want to maintain professional boundaries and not try to influence a patient one way or the other. Sometimes this is difficult because we are so passionate about helping others. However, it is vital to remember that as an advocate you are only providing information and support. Consider for a moment a patient who is a Jehovah's Witness who will not agree to a blood transfusion because it is against his or her religion. What if he or she starts to hemorrhage and the only thing that will save his or her life is a blood transfusion? Although you may really want the patient to give consent you cannot try to persuade the patient. The only thing you and the other health care providers can do is to be sure that the patient understands the risks and benefits of receiving or not receiving this blood transfusion.

Justice is the principle of fair and appropriate treatment. Distributive justice is the fair distribution of goods and services. Thus patients must be treated equally. Using this principle one must question the issue of resources and financial burden. For example, should a patient who abuses drugs and alcohol receive a liver transplant? Or should a 95-year-old who is in fairly good health undergo heart surgery. These are just two examples of ethical dilemmas and as you can see, there is no wrong or right answer. Although some people may feel that neither one of these patients should receive this level of care, others may feel they have the same rights as any other person. What value can someone place on another person's life? This is not an easy question. However, applying ethical principles in daily practice can help nurses and other health care workers to critically think and analyze situations so that they may advocate for the rights of their patients and families.

EXEMPLAR—ARTIFICIAL NUTRITION AND HYDRATION: ETHICAL PERSPECTIVE

During the 1960s, advances in medical technology enabled patients with minimal brain activity to be kept alive with life support. One well-known case is that of Karen Ann Quinlan, which involved the issue of removing her from the ventilator. This led to debates about a patient's right to die and to the legislation regarding living wills. In 1976 California was the first state to approve living wills. Currently, all 50 states have similar legislation. However, the debate regarding withdrawal of life support continues and has been wrought with political and legal conflict (Scroggin, 2007).

The issue about whether to administer, withhold, or withdraw artificial nutrition and hydration has sparked fierce debates in the medical, legal, ethical, and religious arenas. In the past artificial nutrition and hydration (ANH) has been viewed as a medical treatment in which the patient or surrogate had the ability to decide whether or not to allow it. This view was not universal but is well known by medical, ethical, and legal practitioners (Casarett, Kapo, & Caplan, 2005). However, this view has been challenged due in part to well-known legal cases such as the Nancy Cruzan case and the Terri Schiavo case. Nancy Cruzan was a young woman involved in a motor vehicle accident who suffered irreversible brain damage. She was being kept alive with ANH and her parents fought to have it removed because they knew their daughter's wishes. There were several court hearings and overturned decisions and eventually the parents won their case, the gastrostomy tube was removed and Nancy Cruzan died. In Ms. Cruzan's case the family and the health care providers disagreed. However, in the case of Terry Schiavo, a young woman who was in a persistent vegetative state, there was a disagreement between her spouse and parents as to how to proceed with her care. The parents wanted her kept alive and the spouse said they had discussed her wishes and she would not have wanted to be kept alive in this condition. Eventually, the husband won the case, ANH was discontinued and Ms. Schiavo died a few days later (McGowan, 2011). In addition, rising health care costs and a recent papal statement that discourages the withdrawal of ANH in patients who are in a persistent vegetative state have further complicated the issue (Casarett et al, 2005). The Vatican's position views ANH as basic care and not a medical intervention. In March 2004, Pope John Paul II further stated that withdrawal of feeding tubes is "euthanasia by omission" (Scroggin, 2007) However, a majority of American Catholic ethicists and other professionals would not agree with this premise (Jones, 2004). Hence, the issue becomes more complex. It may not be possible to prevent all disagreements regarding this issue but it is essential to "clarify the principles that should underlie decisions about ANH and to ensure that these principles guide decisions in clinical practice" (Jones, 2004, p. 5). The guidelines of the American Academy of Neurology state that ANH is a medical treatment and may be discontinued as it provides no benefit to patients in a persistent vegetative state (Jecker, Jonsen, & Pearlman, 2007). The use of artificial nutrition and hydration can prevent a person's death and is a therapeutic intervention for many patients with various medical conditions. However, its use in patients in a persistent vegetative state may actually cause harm or prolong pain and suffering. ANH can be administered peripherally or enterally. The enteral procedure involves an informed consent, physician order, insertion of a nasogastric or gastrostomy tube, fluoroscopy to verify placement, nutritional consultation, and administration of an enteral feeding. The risk involved in this procedure includes aspiration pneumonia, diarrhea, abdominal discomfort, and may require the patient to be restrained. The life of a patient in a persistent vegetative state may be prolonged up to 10 years, but when ANH is withdrawn the patient will usually die within several days (Casarett, Kapo, & Caplan, 2005). ANH may be viewed as an act of beneficence as the patient's sanctity of life is being maintained. The sanctity-of-life doctrine states, "All human life has worth and therefore it is wrong to take steps to end a person's life, directly or indirectly, no matter what the quality of life" (UK Clinical Ethics Network, 2007, p. 1).

However, this does not take into consideration the pain and suffering of the patient or the patient's family. One must question the rigidity of this doctrine and its ethical implications, as it prevents autonomous decision making and leaves little room for debate.

The Patient Self-Determination Act requires medical institutions to provide information to patients regarding their rights in medical care decisions. These rights include advance directives and the right to refuse treatments. In accordance with the ANA nurses are responsible for implementing and supporting patients' advance directives, especially in end-of-life decisions. Discussions regarding end-of-life care decisions should occur on a routine basis while the patient is still healthy and has the capacity to make his or her wishes known (Burkhart & Nathaniel, 2002). Patients should also be encouraged to make living wills and choose a health care agent who will be familiar with their beliefs regarding end-of-life care. A family discussion should take place to avoid disagreements at times of terminal illness when emotions run high. In the case of Terri Schiavo there was no living will and her parents and her husband had a lengthy legal battle regarding her wishes and whether or not to remove the feeding tube. In the end the court ruled in the husband's favor when that stated his wife would not want to be kept alive in this manner.

The principle of autonomy in a patient who is in a persistent or permanent vegetative state is applicable before the patient becomes incompetent to make decisions. The patient has the right to make choices about his or her life. As stated in Beauchamp and Childress (2001), "Virtually all theories of autonomy agree that two conditions are essential for autonomy: (1) *liberty* (independence from controlling influences) and (2) *agency* (capacity for intentional action)" (p. 58). A living will or durable power of attorney can protect the autonomy of the patient. It is not foolproof and can be burdensome to the person who has been appointed surrogate. Once confronted with the imminent death of a close friend or relative the person may be ambivalent and feel morally responsible for causing the patient's death. The designee now has the autonomy to make life-saving or life-ending decisions, which may be complicated by disagreement of other family members. There may also be disagreement on the part of the health care team. If the health care team feels ANH is not therapeutic or causing harm to the patient they can seek approval for discontinuation of treatment. The issue will be addressed initially by the ethics committee at the health care facility and may be escalated into the legal arena if both sides continue to disagree. At all times the patient's best interest should be the main priority in making such painful decisions. When a patient's wishes are not known, and in the absence of an assigned health care agent, the health care team should collaborate with the patient's surrogate to choose what a reasonable person would choose. "The Uniform Health-Care Decisions Act achieves most of these aims in a clear and thoughtful way and should be adopted by state legislatures" (Casarett et al., 2005, p. 2610). Most states have adopted some form of this act, however, a living will and assigning a durable power of attorney are highly recommended to avoid confusion and lengthy court proceedings. This act gives the surrogate power to withdraw ANH even if the patient's wishes are unknown.

The use of artificial nutrition and hydration has risks and benefits to the patient. There remains a lack of understanding and conflicting views regarding this issue. The benefit to the patient is prolonged life; but at what cost? When the patient is in a persistent vegetative state there is slim, if any, chance of recovery, barring a miracle. With advancing technology this could change. Some people believe that a cure or medical intervention may be developed that will eventually save a person's life and therefore they want to do everything in their power to keep their loved one alive. The family may benefit by avoiding the death of a loved one and savor the time spent with the patient. It is also difficult to think of a loved one being starved to death. It sounds painful and tortuous. However, current literature states that neither nutrition nor hydration increase comfort or quality of life. Research indicates that physiological adaptation will prevent suffering of patients in the withdrawal of ANH (ADA, 2007). Palliative care can be used to promote the comfort of the dying patient whose body begins to shut down and feedings, while absorbed, will fail to nourish. The risks of ANH are well known and must be considered in regard to the principle of non maleficence. This principle of non maleficence mandates health care practitioners to avoid harm. This includes harm that may occur to the patient during acts that are deemed beneficent (Burkhart & Nathaniel, 2002). The use of artificial nutrition is associated with multiple risks to the patient and questionable benefits. Death may be viewed as an end to suffering and therefore an act of beneficence.

The doctrine of double effect distinguishes intentions related to a patient's death. One is the intention to cause death and the other is an act that may result in death, which is an unintended consequence. It is an action with a possible good or bad effect but the act itself is done with the intention of achieving a good effect. Therefore, the act of withdrawing ANH would not be viewed as having a negative effect even if it resulted in the death of the patient (Allmark, 2010). However, some may view withdrawal as negative—thus the doctrine would not be applicable.

Patients and families must have meaningful discussions with clinicians to facilitate the process of informed consent. The medical, legal, and ethical aspects as well as the risks and benefits must be discussed. "Informed consent provides legal protection of a patient's right to personal autonomy"(Burkhardt & Nathaniel, 2002, p. 209). The patient or patient's surrogate is given the opportunity to make an autonomous choice regarding consent to procedures, treatments, and refusal of such procedures. A patient should be given the opportunity to make informed end-of-life care decisions while still healthy.

Justice is the principle of fair and appropriate treatment. Distributive justice is the fair distribution of goods and services. Thus patients must be treated equally. Using this theory one must question the issue of resources and financial burden. A patient in a persistent vegetative state requires expensive medical and nursing care. The patient may be kept alive for many years with no quality of life and little chance of recovery. Financial issues may influence decisions made by hospital administrators and insurance companies. Despite the family/health care agents' wishes to keep their loved one alive by ANH they may decide the cost is too high and challenge the rights of the patient to continue to receive this lifesaving treatment. Distributive justice theory may apply in this type of scenario. Therefore, based on this type of ethical reasoning, some might be of the belief that monies should be directed at patients who have the potential to recover. This is just one example of a possible ethical issue you may face during your nursing career. Because of the complexity of ethical dilemmas they are subject to review by your organization's ethics committee. As you can see there is no right or wrong side and each ethical issue must be analyzed on an individual case-by-case basis. The ethics committee must look at both sides of the issue and make a determination using the ethical principles and first and foremost consider the best interest and wishes, if known, of the patient. When the hospital and the patient's family or health care agent do not agree the ethical committee will be convened. If they cannot come to consensus either party may seek legal counsel.

MORAL ISSUES

Nurses also face many moral issues in their day-to-day practice and although one's morals are usually developed throughout one's life there are different theories that describe moral development. For example, Gilligan's theory of moral reasoning was developed in response to the cognitive developmental stage theory of moral development proposed by Kohlberg (Jaffe & Hyde, 2000). Kohlberg's theory involves six stages of moral development that are based on Piaget's stages of moral judgment. The six stages include: obedience and punishment orientation, individualism and exchange, cognitive good interpersonal relationships, maintaining the social order, social contract and individual rights, and universal principles. The learner develops and achieves these stages as she or he advances through her or his academic development (Bastable, 2003: Kretchmar, 2008, as cited in Hunt, 2013). Gilligan challenged Kohlberg's research, which was understood to be gender biased, as his subjects were all male. Gilligan (1982) challenged prior theories of moral development and looked at it from a broader perspective, which included a care orientation and a justice orientation theory. She further theorized that most females use the care perspective and most males use the justice perspective. Beauchamp and Childress (2001) posit that "male subjects typically view morality in terms of rights and justice" (p. 370). The caring perspective is very different from the justice perspective in that personal feelings are involved in the decision. There is a strong emotional component, which cannot be ignored. "The care orientation is characterized by a focus on maintaining relationships, responding to the needs of others, and a responsibility not to cause hurt" (Jaffe & Hyde, 2000, p. 2). "Care ethics also casts care as either a challenge to the masculinism of theoretical conceptions of justice, in what is framed in terms of the 'care vs. justice' debate" (Gilligan et al., 1982, as cited in Cloyes, 2002). "The justice orientation is concerned with principles of fairness and equity such as those assessed in conventional moral reasoning" (Gilligan, 1982, p. 75). Caring is a difficult concept to measure and the ability to care varies among all individuals. Moral values also vary based on past and present development in addition to cultural influences. Moral development begins in childhood when children learn right from wrong and continues into adulthood as adults gain better insight into their actions. Moral issues faced by the nurse involve more than knowing "right" from "wrong" as health care is complex and there are always confounding issues that require careful analysis and thought. For example, based on religious or cultural beliefs a nurse may feel that a DNR order is morally wrong. However, he or she has a moral obligation to honor the patient's wishes. It is helpful to complete a self-assessment of your cultural beliefs, values, and practices so you identify areas that may prove to be morally challenging. There are also options available to nurses who would find it morally unacceptable to partake in certain practices. Abortion is one of those practices in which nurses have the right to refuse to participate. No one can tell you how to think or feel but being a nurse will at times challenge your morals.

LEGAL ISSUES

Laws are developed to protect people from harm and it is very important to understand the legalities of health care and the nursing profession. To practice nursing one must complete a program of study, pass a licensure exam, and maintain current licensure in any state in which one chooses to practice. Nurses are legally bound to this process and to follow the Nurse Practice Act (see Chapter 1). Nurses must consider multiple legal issues that may occur in their daily practice. These issues relate to their personal practice and the nursing care they provide to their patients. "In order to effectively advocate on behalf of patients and protect them from medical errors, nurses must understand the patient's legal rights and advocate for those rights to multidisciplinary members of the health care team" (Priest et al., 2007, p. 35.). Our society is becoming more litigious and students and nurses must be aware of this situation. According to Klaassen et al. (2011), legal and disciplinary actions against nurses are on the rise; between 1997 and 2007, insurance payouts for judgments of $10,000 or more against registered nurses almost doubled in number and equaled more than $94 million. Furthermore, student nurses also face legal issues related to alcohol, substance abuse, and psychiatric issues that may prevent them from taking their licensure exams. Although guidelines have been developed by the American Nurses Association (ANA) and the American Association of Colleges of Nurses (AACN), many students do not understand the full ramifications of the legal and ethical issues that impact their profession. To address this pervasive issue, The American Association of Nurse Attorneys had developed a comprehensive curriculum for faculty to follow when teaching students about legal issues. If your school does not provide this information it is imperative that you take control of your knowledge acquisition and explore ways to learn more about these issues. For example, you may read the literature and attend continuing-education courses or seminars on these topics.

Legal issues relate to the following areas:

- Following hospital policy
- Scope of practice
- Safe medication administration
- Provision of care
- Competency
- Documentation
- Reporting errors
- Insubordination
- Patient abandonment

- HIPAA (Health Insurance Portability and Accountability Act) violations
- Substance abuse and working while impaired
- Patient advocacy
- End-of-life issues

Pappas et al. (2007) recommend that the following legal modules/topics, which have been developed with input from a nurse attorney, be included in all nursing programs:

- Care of emancipated minor
- Hospital lawsuits
- Nurse malpractice and the attorney
- Liability of nurse managers
- Physician's orders
- Nursing charting and technology
- End-of-life authorizations

Emancipated Minor

An emancipated minor is person who is under the age of 18 but due to circumstances he or she can legally make decisions and give informed consent for treatment. An example of an emancipated minor is a 16-year-old female who has given birth to a child. According to Schwabb and Pohlman (2002), although state laws vary, an individual who is pregnant, a parent, or in the military is considered an emancipated minor.

It is important to ascertain the status of a minor when obtaining informed consent for treatment. Keep in mind that there are regulations for consents and you will need to follow your hospital's policy. For example, in general all invasive procedures require an informed written consent, whereas many noninvasive treatments, such as medication administration or dressing changes, require a verbal assent. Furthermore, on admission patients or surrogates sign a general-consent-to-treatment form but this does not pertain to invasive procedures.

Hospital Lawsuits and Malpractice

Lawsuits and claims relating to negligence and malpractice are something we certainly hope never happen. Unfortunately, we all must be prepared because there is a high probability that throughout one's academic or professional journey one may be involved in a lawsuit.

This could be as a witness or as the person who engaged in negligence and/or malpractice. This is why it is imperative for students and nurses to purchase their own malpractice insurance. Even though you may be covered by your organization's insurance it is important to also have your own.

In a malpractice case, a patient's lawyer must prove that:

1. A nurse had a duty to a patient
2. The duty was breached
3. The patient was injured
4. The injury was caused by the breach of duty (Moniz, 1996, p. 45)

The best way to avoid a malpractice case is to follow your Nurse Practice Act along with your hospital's policies and procedures, standards of care, and clinical practice guidelines, and to use evidence-based practice. It is also vital to complete your documentation as per hospital policy and legal guidelines. Nurses must know when to consult with their superiors about an issue, and it is also important to escalate issues and inform your supervisor of potential problems. When in doubt about anything you should consult with your nurse manager or supervisor for guidance on how to proceed. If you do have the misfortune to be involved in a legal case you should notify your malpractice carrier, who will then advise you on what actions are required. Your legal counsel will help you to prepare for legal hearings. Many cases are settled out of court and some are frivolous and are dismissed very quickly. One does not want to become paralyzed with fear when providing care to patients, however, an "ounce of prevention is worth a pound of cure" so it is best to be prepared for all possibilities, both positive and negative.

Documentation

Documentation and integrity of medical records, whether they are in electronic format or in a chart, is another important responsibility of nurses and other health care providers.

Although health care organizations use various methods and have specific guidelines related to documentation, organizations also share similarities. For example, there are the legalities of documentation and standards set forth by various private and public, local, state, and government agencies. "Documentation of patient care is a critical skill used by nurses to communicate patient care, assess and record patients' progress and provide evidence of not only care given and patients' responses but also an evaluation of care given (Aitken et al., 2006; Cheevakasemsook et al., 2006; as cited in Tower et al., 2012, p. 2918). Tower et al. (2012) point out that despite widespread agreement that nursing documentation should be a chronological account that accurately reflects the care provided to the patient, there are significant deficiencies in documentation that may result in adverse patient outcome. Therefore, it is vitally important to follow your organization's policies and procedures for documentation; however, one must also be knowledgeable about the legal and ethical implications that apply. The patient's medical record is a legal document and anything that is added becomes part and parcel of the record. For example, one is not allowed to erase, cross out, change, add, or remove documents. In the event of an error one can place one line through a handwritten entry, identify this as an error and place your initials over the sentence or words. An addendum may also be added at a later point in time as long as it is clearly identified as an addendum with the date and time of entry. You also need to be careful not to make assumptions. You need to include objective and subjective data that are based on your assessment findings. For example, if a patient's body language is suggesting that he or she is depressed you should not document that the patient is depressed (medical dx) but state what you are observing (e.g., patient is crying with head downcast). Electronic medical records are somewhat different; however, the same legal principles apply. Following the steps of the nursing process can be very helpful when documenting and organizing your notes. Assessment is always a priority and your findings should be included in your documentation. This may be in the form of a checklist or written in narrative form based on your organization's policies. When you begin a new clinical rotation as a student or a new position as a nurse you will be taught about the specific forms and requirements for documentation as per the organization. Once you assess your patient you need to decide on your next course of action. This will depend on the situation. If the patient is having difficulty your plan and intervention may be to notify the health care provider or administer a stat treatment. Whatever the case you will want to outline specific interventions and evaluate the patient's response to treatment. At this point you may need to continue or revise your plan and interventions. The caveat being there should be no open circles or dangling participles, if you will. It is not enough to document the problem or issue, you must also document what you did and whether or not it was effective.

Exemplar

Mrs. G is a 42-year-old female with diverticulitis who is 12 hours post a colon resection. She is reporting a pain level of eight in her abdominal area. You immediately conduct an assessment of her pain using the PQRST method: P = provoking symptoms, Q = quality of pain, R = radiation, S = severity, T = timing and duration. You assess her vitals and check her orders for as needed pain medications. You also check when the last time she received the pain medication was. If her vitals are stable and she is due to receive her pain medication (e.g., morphine 3 mg intravenously), you verify the order, obtain the medication, return to patient's room, wash your hands, verify patient identification, follow the six rights of medication administration, and document the administration of the medication in the appropriate place. You also document this in the patient's medical record in either narrative form or using a checklist. You will then continue to monitor your patient's response to this treatment and reassess her as per hospital policy. If the patient is stable and reports that her pain level is decreasing you document the findings and continue to monitor. If the patient's pain is worse or her vital signs are unstable you will need to contact the licensed provider and revise your plan of care. All of this should be documented in the medical record. If the patient is stable when you assess her it is important to demonstrate that you are monitoring your patient throughout the shift.

Documentation should also include your plan of care, patient education, discharge planning, and any issues that may arise throughout your shift. Not only are your notes vital to promoting positive outcomes, they also demonstrate that you were not negligent in your responsibilities and that you followed standards of care and practice. Furthermore, if perchance you are involved with a lawsuit your notes will be helpful to you because it is difficult to recall something that occurred several years ago. Due to the nature of lawsuits, you may be called either as a witness or defendant several years after you cared for a particular patient. If you have detailed documentation it will prove quite helpful to you and your legal counsel. Tower et al. (2012) examined situational awareness and decision-making processes of registered nurses while documenting. They suggest that improving situational awareness and developing a decision-making model could be instrumental in improving nursing documentation.

Abandonment and Insubordination

The professional practice role entails major responsibilities to your patients, organization, and profession. There are times when you may feel that you have been given an unfair assignment and although you may be correct you must remember that you have an obligation to your patients. However, you need to be aware that if you refuse the assignment you may be charged with abandonment or insubordination. Furthermore, there are channels and a chain of command you must follow. States have different definitions of what constitutes abandonment so it is important to know your state's regulations (Blyth, 2007). "If a claim for patient abandonment is substantiated, the nurse's license to practice may be suspended" (Blyth, 2007, p. 8). Wilson and Commons (2008) posit that not all refusals to complete an assignment are considered abandonment, especially if said assignment would put a patient at risk of harm. However, leaving your assigned unit without notifying the supervisor and waiting for coverage, leaving for personal reasons (e.g., going outside to smoke), or leaving for any reason without transferring care to another nurse may be considered abandonment. You work hard to obtain your RN license and do not want to do anything that may result in harm to your patients or loss of your license so be sure to follow proper protocol when any issues arise relating to your ability to safely care for your patients.

Insubordination is another serious issue that may have a negative effect on your employment and may result in disciplinary actions and charges of misconduct. "Insubordination is the refusal by an employee to obey a lawful and reasonable instruction from his superior" (Motsepe, 2011, p. 40). The key here is that it must be lawful and within your scope of practice. For example, your supervisor may assign you to float to the operating room, which would be highly unlikely. However, if you refuse to go because you did not have the competency and skill sets required to work in this type of unit, you would not be guilty of insubordination. However, even if the idea is as ludicrous as this example, you should still follow your chain of command. According to Motsepe (2011), disrespectful behaviors, such as cursing, are identified as insolence, and not the same as insubordination, albeit they often occur simultaneously. Employees who are insubordinate may be guilty of misconduct and be terminated from their place of employment. An employee who is insolent will most likely be disciplined; however, he or she will not be terminated unless the employee has a pattern of this type of unprofessional behavior.

Professional boundaries relate to the space between the power of the nurse and the vulnerability of the patient. Nurses must establish boundaries with patients to balance power and ensure safe interactions. It is also vital to prevent violations of boundaries, which includes too little or too much involvement while delivering patient-centered care, with the most grievous being sexual misconduct (National Council of State Boards of Nursing [NCSBN], 2011). According to the NCSBN (2011) the following are examples of violations of professional boundaries:

- Excessive self-disclosure
- Secretive behavior
- Super-nurse behavior
- Singled-outpatient treatment
- Flirtations
- You-and-me-against-the-world behavior
- Failure to protect the patient

These violations may be inadvertent or purposeful and must be avoided at all costs. Furthermore, nurses must also report violations made by other members of the health care team.

End-of-Life Care

End-of-life care has major legal implications for nurses who are in the prime position as patient advocates assisting patients, families, and surrogates to understand the options for end of life. According to McGowan (2011) critical care nurses play a vital role in end-of-life dilemmas such as assessing patients' mental capacity and assisting families and/or surrogates to make decisions regarding such things as removal from a ventilator in a patient who is in a persistent vegetative state. Many end-of-life dilemmas are resolved within the hospital setting; however, some are resolved in the court system, such as the Schiavo and Cruzan cases (McGlown, 2011). These cases are quite difficult and fraught with emotions; acceptance of a loved one's passing, even when things seem hopeless, is something we hope never to have to experience. Although the experience is different for nurses and other health care providers who are not as emotionally involved, end-of-life care requires caring, empathy, and moral, ethical, and legal decision making. It can be difficult to separate one's personal beliefs from what is right and just especially when there is no right or wrong decision. However, at the end of the day we need to know that we advocated for our patients based on what we believed was in their best interest and based on their wishes. It is imperative that you are aware of your patient's wishes regarding end-of-life care, palliation, and advance directives. For example, you must know whether a patient has a DNR order so that you do not mistakenly administer life-saving therapies. Similarly, you don't want to fail to implement lifesaving measures if a patient does not have a DNR order. On admission this information should be obtained and competent patients should be asked about advance directives and be given an opportunity to make decisions while they are still able. Regulations and laws vary among states and countries so be sure to follow the proper procedures.

TECHNOLOGY AND SOCIAL MEDIA: ETHICAL, LEGAL, AND MORAL IMPLICATIONS

The use of social media has increased exponentially in the past decade and many academic and health care organizations have not been able to foresee and forecast all the potential issues that may arise from this popular form of communication. There have been positive and negative issues related to social media and one must be cognizant of the potential harmful effects of technology and social media. Social media includes websites such as LinkedIn, Twitter, and Facebook, in addition to multiple other websites. Nurses and other health care providers may inadvertently breach patient confidentiality by posting pictures or patient information. "Therefore, prior to engaging in social media platforms all nurses should clearly understand the Health Insurance Portability and Accountability Act (HIPAA) and how to avoid possible privacy ethical violations" (Lachman, 2013, p. 326). The Health Insurance Portability and Accountability Act was passed in 1996 (Foster, 2012, p. 37). HIPAA relates to patient privacy, confidentiality, and protection of patient information (Foster, 2012). Nurses and other health care workers must do everything in their power to maintain patient privacy. It is vital to log off computers, never share passwords, and refrain from discussing patient cases in hallways, elevators, outside of the hospital, or on social media. As a student you will most likely be completing clinical assignments and it is important to only share patients' initials and exclude any identifiers that could be associated with a particular patient. There are times as a student or a nurse when you may care for someone who you know either personally or through a friend or relative. If this happens you must be very careful not to mention this to anyone and not to share any type of information about this patient. Remember HIPAA violations may result in monetary fines and jail time, so there is no room for error. All employees and students complete HIPAA training so you will learn more about this in your clinical courses and later in your professional role. It is better to err on the side of caution and refrain from posting information about patients or issues that occur in the workplace. Although you may want to share an interesting case with your peers, it is best not to do so on social media.

One must also be careful not to disparage one's place of employment, administrators, or colleagues in a public forum. Making disparaging comments against a co worker can be viewed as lateral bullying, which is a breach of the Nurses Code of Ethics. Because of the pervasive nature of the use of social media the American Nurses Association has developed six principles and the National State Boards of Nursing have developed guidelines to help nurses engage in professional use of social media and avoid harm to patients (Lachman, 2013). Some situations are quite innocent and well intentioned but may still involve a breach of confidentiality.

Cell phones have been at the core of multiple issues and many hospitals and health care organizations have policies forbidding their use in clinical areas. Other hospitals allow their employees to use cell phones. In fact, some use them to communicate with their staff nurses on the unit. There are many types of hand-held devices that can be used in the health care setting as a means of researching and locating data in a very efficient manner. However, confidentiality may be breached if employees use their cell phones or other devices to take pictures of patients and/or their medical records. Therefore, it is imperative to know and follow your organization's polices. Furthermore, even if cell phones are allowed there are still restrictions on their use. For example, unless it is a requirement of one's position, cell phones should not be used at the patient's bedside or anywhere in the unit. And you should never take pictures of patients or visitors with your cell phone or any other hand-held device. Because all organizations have different policies you should become well versed in the accepted policy. HIPPA violations are very serious and are punishable by law with possible fines and jail time so it is imperative to protect our patients' personal information at all times.

SUMMARY

This chapter presented an overview of legal, ethical, and moral issues that are faced by nurses and other health care professionals. It is important to have a basic understanding of how these issues inform practice. Furthermore, because of differences in local, state, national, and global laws and standards, one must be cognizant of the specific laws that influence his or her practice. These issues are quite complex and require more in-depth exploration.

Discussion Questions

1. Identify three ethical issues that may occur in the hospital setting.
2. List and describe the ethical principles that are applied when analyzing an ethical issue.
3. What is utilitarianism?
4. Identify three legal issues that impact your role as a registered nurse.
5. Discuss HIPAA and its significance.
6. Describe Kohlberg's theory of moral development.
7. What constitutes abandonment?
8. What are some taboos when documenting?
9. Who would be considered an emancipated minor?
10. What is an informed consent?

Suggested Learning Activities

- Role-play various legal, moral, and ethical scenarios.
- Select an ethical issue and write an essay demonstrating both sides of the issue.
- Complete a review of the literature on the legalities of documentation and write a three-page essay.
- Interview a lawyer about legal issues that inform nursing practice.
- Interview an ethicist.

REFERENCES

Allmark, P., Cobb, M., Liddle, B., & Tod, A. (2010). Is the doctrine of double effect irrelevant in end-of-life decision making? *Nursing Philosophy, 11*(3), 170–177. doi:10.1111/j.1466-769X.2009.00430.x

American Dietetic Association. (2007). *Ethical and legal issues in nutrition, hydration and feeding.* Retrieved from http://Public/Nutrition Information/92_8330 .cfm

American Nurses Association (ANA). (2011). *ANA's principles for social networking and the nurse.* Silver Spring, MD: Author.

Arries, E. (2014). Patient safety and quality in healthcare: Nursing ethics for ethics quality. *Nursing Ethics, 21*(1), 3–5. doi:10.1177/0969733013509042

Aitken, R., Manias, E., & Dunning, T. (2006). Documentation of medication management by graduate nurses in patient progress notes: a way forward for patient safety. *Collegian, 13*, 5–11.

Beauchamp, T., & Childress, J. (2001). *Principles of biomedical ethics* (5th ed.). New York, NY: Oxford University Press.

Blyth, D. (2007). Do you know what constitutes patient abandonment? *Nursing Management, 38*(8), 8.

Burkhardt, M., & Nathaniel, A. (2013). *Ethics & issues in contemporary nursing* (4th ed.). Stamford, CT: Cengage Learning.

Casarett, D., Kapo, J., & Caplan, A. (2005). Appropriate use of artificial nutrition and hydration—Fundamental principles and recommendations. *New England Journal of Medicine, 353*(24), 2607–2615.

Cheevakasemsook, A., Chapman, Y., Francis, K., & Davis, C. (2006) The study of nursing documentation complexities. *International Journal of Nursing Practice, 12*, 366–374.

Cloyes, K. (2002). Agonizing care: Care ethics, agonistic feminism and a political theory of care. *Nursing Inquiry, 9*(3), 203–214.

Foster, C. (2012). Advocates of privacy. HIPPA 101. *Washington Nurse, 42*(3), 37.

Gilligan, C. (1982). *In a different voice: Psychological theory and women's development.* Cambridge, MA: Harvard University Press.

Harding, T. (2013). Cultural safety: A vital element for nursing ethics. *Nursing Praxis In New Zealand, 29*(1), 4–11.

Jaffe, S., & Hyde, J. S. (2000) Gender differences in moral orientation: A meta-analysis. *Psychological Bulletin, 126*(5), 703–726.

Jecker, N., Jonsen, A., & Pearlman, R. (2007). *Bioethics: An introduction to the history, methods, and practice.* Sudbury, MA: Jones & Bartlett.

Jones, A. (2004, March 26). US ethicists counter Vatican view. *National Catholic Reporter*, p. 5.

Kangasniemi, M., Vaismoradi, M., Jasper, M., & Turunen, H. (2013). Ethical issues in patient safety: Implications for nursing management. *Nursing Ethics, 20*(8), 904–916. doi:10.1177/0969733013484488

Klaassen, J., Smith, K. V., & Witt, J. (2011). The new nexus: Legal concept instruction to nursing students, teaching–learning frameworks, and high fidelity human simulation. *Journal of Nursing Law, 14*(3–4), 85-90. doi:10.1891/1073-7472.14.3.4.85

Lachman, V. D. (2013). Social media: Managing the ethical issues. *Med–Surg Matters, 22*(5), 326–329.

McGowan, C. M. (2011). Legal issues. Legal aspects of end-of-life care. *Critical Care Nurse, 31*(5), 64–69. doi:10.4037/ccn2011550

Moniz, D. (1996). When things go wrong… malpractice lawsuits. *Nursing, 26*(2), 45.

Motsepe, P. (2011). A simple request. *Nursing Update, 35*(7), 40–41.

National Council of State Boards of Nursing. (2011). *A nurse's guide to professional boundaries.* Retrieved from https://www.ncsbn.org/ProfessionalBoundaries

Pappas, I., Clutter, L., & Maggi, E. (2007). Current legal changes: Innovative legal seminar for nursing students. *Journal of Nursing Law, 11*(4), 197–209.

Priest, C., Kooken, W., Ealey, K., Holmes, S., & Hufeld, P. (2007). Improving baccalaureate nursing students' understanding of fundamental legal issues through interdisciplinary collaboration. *Journal of Nursing Law, 11*(1), 35–42.

Schwabb, N., & Pohlman, K. (2002). Legal and ethical issues. Legal and ethical issues: Questions and answers. *Journal of School Nursing, 18*(5), 301–305. doi: 10.1177/10598405020180051001

Scroggin, J. (2007). Planning for medical decisions. *Advisor Today.* Accessed from http://www.advisor.today.com/resources/planmedidecision.htm

Tower, M., Chaboyer, W., Green, Q., Dyer, K., & Wallis, M. (2012). Registered nurses' decision-making regarding documentation in patients' progress notes. *Journal of Clinical Nursing, 21*(19/20), 2917–2929. doi:10.1111/j.1365-2702.2012.04135.x

UK Clinical Ethics Network. (n.d.). *Ethical issues—End of life decisions.* Retrieved from www.ukcen.net

Wilson, B., & Commons, K. (2008). You asked. What is client abandonment? *Nursing BC, 40*(3), 12–13.

PART II

The Path From Graduation to NCLEX Success and First Nursing Position

CHAPTER 7

The Path to NCLEX Success

Nothing will work unless you do.

—Maya Angelou

OBJECTIVES

After reading this chapter, the reader will be able to:

- Discuss ways to prepare for the National Council Licensure Examination for Registered Nurses (NCLEX-RN®)
- Understand the NCLEX plan
- Identify relationship of Bloom's taxonomy to NCLEX
- Understand importance of NCLEX prep
- Identify key aspects in applying for NCLEX
- Develop a contingency plan for retaking the NCLEX

The path to NCLEX success certainly begins when you enter nursing school. However, in actuality it begins much earlier because all of the knowledge and experience you have garnered throughout your formal and informal education will be invaluable as you navigate your way through your formal nursing program. Passing the NCLEX and transitioning into your role as a professional nurse requires synthesis of theoretical concepts and course content from all of your coursework. You will also need to be able to critically think and reason, prioritize, and problem solve. Sometimes students don't understand the significance of the foundational courses they complete. However, if you consider math and science as the building blocks for your nursing curriculum you will real-ize their importance. Many students cram and memorize facts so they can pass a class, but never really understand the material. However, if you want to be successful you need to retain the information. For example, although you are not becoming a pharmacist you still need to understand chemistry and physiology so you know what effect the medications you administer to your patients will have on their systems. The nursing cur-riculum is carefully developed with courses and content that are vital to your role as a nurse. Of course, it is impossible to remember every fact and that is why you must commit to being a lifelong learner.

Learning how to become a nurse is so much more than passing a licensure exam, it is everything before, during, and after formal educa-tion that helps you to develop as a nurse. And it is important to realize that this is a journey that will continue throughout your entire profes-sional career. One might question why he or she has to take a review class or spend so many hours preparing for the NCLEX after spending so much time learning and studying in school. Review classes are not mandatory, however, they do help you to respond to the type of ques-tions you will be expected to answer on your NCLEX exam. Nursing school prepares one to be a novice nurse generalist, and while you are prepared to take the NCLEX, the focus is much broader in scope and your faculty would be doing a disservice to you if they only taught you what was going to be on the exam.

LICENSING EXAMS

All countries have specific program and licensing requirements for registered nurses. Although these differ among geographic areas they share the common goal of developing a standardized way to evaluate whether a candidate possesses the basic knowledge required to prac-tice as a registered nurse. "The measure of student success addressed in most literature is the National Council Licensure Examination (NCLEX) passing rates" (Sewell et al., 2008, p. 109). The National Council of State Boards of Nurses (NCSBN) is an organization that collaborates with individual state boards of nursing in the development of the NCLEX with the overarching goal of public health and safety (NCSBN, 2014). The National Council of State Boards of Nursing is comprised of del-egates from each state in the United States, several U.S. territories, and 16 associate members from other countries.

Individual states have their own state boards that oversee licens-ing and registration of nurses and other licensed personnel. Each state has delegates on the National Council of State Boards of Nursing and therefore have input into the NCLEX and its development. Because there is one national exam nurses who wish to work in other states do not need to take a new exam; however, they do need to apply for registration through reciprocity. Nurses qualified outside the United States who plan to practice in the United States must take the Commission on Graduates of Foreign Nursing Schools (CGFNS) examination ("Nursing in the U.S.," 2014). Each country has its own requirements and it is important for you to understand these requirements so that you can prepare for your exam. If you are licensed in the United States and you wish to work in another country you will most likely need to take that particular country's licensing exam. Your nursing school should be able to give you information and guidance as you prepare to take your exam. Your school administrator must also certify that you have successfully completed all the requirements of the nursing program.

NCLEX-RN®

The National Council Licensure Examination is the exam that is taken by nurses in the United States. According to Aucoin and Treas (2005), state licensing agencies and state accrediting bodies use performance on the NCLEX as a primary measure of program achievement. "To ensure public protection, NCSBN member board jurisdictions require a candidate for licensure to pass an exam that measures the competencies needed to perform safely and effectively as a newly licensed, entry-level nurse" (NCSBN, 2014). The NCLEX is currently offered as a computerized multiple-choice exam and candidates may be required to answer anywhere from 75 to 265 questions in a 6-hour period. The type of program used is Computerized Adaptive Testing (CAT) and it responds to your individual responses. When you answer a question the computer re-estimates your ability and adjusts the difficulty of the question to better match your ability. Every time you answer a question the computer becomes more precise in estimating your ability. The questions are designed to be challenging and you have a 50% chance of answering each item correctly (NCSBN, 2014).

Every 3 years the test plan is updated and revised. The test plan is readily available on the NCSBN's website so it is highly recommended that you review the information about the NCLEX test plan. Furthermore, there is a wealth of other helpful information on this site. The questions on NCLEX are based on Bloom's higher order domains of application and analysis. Bloom's taxonomy will be discussed in greater detail later in this chapter. The framework is based on clients' needs and is divided into several categories. According to the NCLEX test plan the following categories are included on NCLEX:

- Safe and effective care environment
- Management of care
- Safety and infection control
- Health promotion and maintenance
- Psychosocial integrity
- Physiological integrity
- Basic care and comfort
- Pharmacological and parenteral therapies
- Reduction of risk potential
- Physiological adaptation

Throughout the exam the following integrated processes that are fundamental to nursing are woven into each question: nursing process, caring, communication/documentation, and teaching/learning. There is a specific formula relating to distribution of content and an overview of specific content is provided in the NCLEX test plan, located on the NCSBN's website. There is also information about the specific categories and some sample questions. This information will be most beneficial to you as you are preparing for the exam.

Applying for NCLEX is a multistep process that requires collaboration with your school administration. Before applying for NCLEX you should develop a plan outlining your preparation with dates for when you plan to take the exam. Keep in mind that although you may have graduated your school needs to complete a review prior to certifying that you have met all the requirements of the program and are eligible to sit for the exam. You can consult your individual state or country's (outside of the U.S.) licensing board for directions on how to apply and schedule your exam. In the United States, each candidate contacts her or his licensing board and applies for registration and must supply the correct personal identification and pay the required fee. When the Board of Nursing verifies that you meet all the requirements you will be given Authorization to Test (ATT). Once you are authorized you will have approximately 90 days to schedule your exam. As you can see this requires careful planning and thought. Studies demonstrate that the ideal time to take the NCLEX is within 3 months of graduating (Lavin & Rosario-Sim, 2013). Developing a clear plan for preparing and taking the exam is crucial. Bonis, Taft, and Wendler (2007) recommend the following:

- Accept responsibility for success on the NCLEX-RN.
- Develop a specific study plan.
- Use review courses, review books, and CDs.
- Use practice questions and practice tests.
- Engage in stress management (p. 86).

You also want to have a contingency plan just in case you need to retake the exam. You also need to consider whether or not you qualify for testing accommodations. If you have been receiving accommodations in school, such as extended testing time, then you should probably explore your options. Many students who were eligible for testing accommodations but did not apply for them do so the second time and then pass the NCLEX. You are the best judge of what your learning needs are and must self-advocate for whatever accommodations you require.

BLOOM'S TAXONOMY

The six domains developed by Bloom are knowledge, comprehension, application, analysis, synthesis, and evaluation (Anderson, 1994; Bloom, 1956). Dr. Lorin Anderson, a former student of Bloom's, revised the taxonomy to reflect teaching and learning more broadly and in response to advances in education that have taken place since Bloom developed the original taxonomy.

The new terms are remembering (recognizing), understanding (summarizing), applying (implementing), analyzing (differentiating) evaluating (making judgements), and creating (planning or producing) with each domain increasing in complexity and knowledge development. (Anderson & Krathwohl, 2001, as cited in Hunt, 2013).

The domains of learning are used by the developers of the NCLEX exam with most questions at the analysis and application level. Many educators develop their test questions and assessments using these domains. The questions will increase in difficulty as you progress through your program or even throughout the semester. Understanding these domains can help you to prepare for your exams because a "knowledge or remembering" question is quite different from a "synthesis, evaluation, or analysis" question. Many review books and even your textbooks will include different levels of questions based on Bloom's taxonomy. Quite often they will include a rationale, and identify the level of difficulty of a question, and how it relates to the licensure exam.

PREPARING FOR YOUR LICENSING EXAM

It is never too early or too late to prepare for your licensing exam. As previously stated the day you being your nursing program is the day you begin preparing for your exam and your role as a professional nurse. According to Lavendera et al. (2011), "The first–time pass rate for the NCLEX-RN licensure examination has decreased nationally from 79.9% in 1995 to 69.9% in 2008" (NCSBN, 2009). This is a significant drop and the test is becoming more complex so it is certainly in your best interest to be well prepared for this exam. Self-efficacy has been associated with nursing student success and retention (Shelton, 2012). Although the onus is on you as an individual to pass this exam, you will not be alone in your journey. Your faculty will be helping to prepare you for your role as a nurse generalist as you progress through your courses. Part of this preparation will be integrated into all of your courses by your expert faculty who will use a variety of teaching and learning strategies that will guide your knowledge development and enhance your critical-thinking and problem-solving skills.

In at least some of your courses you will be given exams that are similar to the licensure exam with questions that have been developed in accordance with Bloom's taxonomy. These exams serve dual purposes: assessment of learning and preparation for licensure exam. Romeo (2013) examined factors that predict NCLEX success and found that the two most significant predictors of NCLEX success are grade point average (GPA) in nursing courses and scores on standardized exams. Being able to think critically is a key component in this exam—thus emphasizing the significance of doing well in courses and completing exercises that are geared to improving your critical-thinking and reasoning skills. Simon et al. (2013) examined predictors related to success on the National League for Nursing (NLN) Diagnostic Readiness Test (DRT) for RN Licensure and found a positive relationship among GPA, high scores in biology and chemistry, completion of a high-quality nursing foundation course, remediation, and ongoing support and NCLEX success. One study identified admission criteria and course performance as predictors of future success in the nursing licensure exam (Lavendera et al., 2011). The results of these studies demonstrate the significance of preparing for NCLEX throughout your program.

Being an active learner and mastering the content throughout your program will be key components to your NCLEX success and, more importantly, your role as a registered professional nurse. Strategies for NCLEX-RN success include study groups, developing a study plan, taking review courses, test-taking strategies and coaching, time management, use of review books, and using relaxation and anxiety-reduction techniques (Bonis et al., 2007, p.84). Certainly, becoming a nurse is so much more than passing an exam; however, that is the key that grants you entry into practice. Hence it is vital to develop a plan for success. Understanding the relationship between GPA and passing the NCLEX should serve as a motivator to do your best in all of your classes (Raman, 2013). Study groups are extremely helpful throughout your program of study and while preparing for your licensure exam. Developing an informal contract with your study partners can be quite helpful in keeping you all on the same page. A study plan is another vital tool you can use because you can break down the material into smaller parts. This may be done informally or formally, however, a formal group will provide more structure and greater commitment. For example, you might develop a plan (see Table 7.1) and break it down into systems or specific topics and be specific as to goals and objectives and roles and responsibilities. This plan will work for any exam you are preparing to take. Study groups can be very helpful but one must avoid the pitfalls of engaging in too much socialization during the allotted time.

The development of study skills is also a vital component for successful completion of your program of study and your licensure exam. Fischer et al. (2001) identify several areas required for developing good study skills: the ability to find information, the synthesis of information, and the consequent application and integration of information into practice. Many students spend hours preparing for exams but do not do well because they do not know how to study. Many academic organizations provide students with tutoring, support, and seminars to improve study skills, writing, math, and other skills. Individual faculty members may also provide extra help or review classes throughout the semester. Try to take advantage of all the support that is offered by your organization and your mentors.

Many schools use programs that are geared at preparing you for the NCLEX. Certainly if your school has such a program you should take full advantage of every resource available. Homard (2013) found that bachelor of science nursing (BSN) students who completed four semesters of a standardized test package had higher scores and NCLEX pass rates than the students who did not participate in the package. An example of this type of program is the Assessment Technology Institute (ATI), the Health Education Incorporated Systems (HESI) exam by Elsevier,

TABLE 7.1
Study Plan for Med–Surg Exam

Topical Outline: (list all topics to be covered) _____

Purpose of Study Group: (midterm or final exam) _____

Goal: (members should develop a goal) _____

Objectives: (members should develop measurable objectives) _____

Study Strategies: (e.g., reviewing notes, listening to recorded lectures, discussion questions, practice questions, quizzing each other, flashcards, and stress reduction) _____

Members: (list all members) _____

Member Agreement: (members should sign a contract) _____

Member Responsibilities: (notes, practice questions, study guide, role play)
_____

Meeting Dates and Times: (set specific dates and times) _____

Meeting Location: (library, study hall) _____

Post-Test Debriefing: (what worked, what didn't work, how can we improve our group) _____

or a Kaplan course, whereas some students develop their own review courses. The Assessment Technology Institute program helps prepare students for the NCLEX-RN. The program offers education, assessment, and testing. Schools decide the type of program that will best meet their needs. For example, ATI can be used in all the theory/clinical courses with resources and testing at the completion of the course. The test questions are based on the NCLEX-RN plan so are very similar to the type of questions you will complete on the formal NCLEX-RN. Your faculty may assign points for this type of learning activity or it may just be a requirement for the course. There is also a comprehensive test for a senior student that is predictive of NCLEX success. The program offers a variety of resources, such as interactive videos, non proctored exams, and content-specific remediation that is based on the individual's test scores and learning needs (ATI, 2014). In some states the ATI or similar exam is used for progression from one level to the next; however, states, such as New York, do not allow standardized tests to prevent a student from progressing to the next level.

There are many review classes available to you when you graduate that will help you prepare for your licensure exam. It is not mandatory to take one of these courses, but many students find them helpful. Some have guarantees so in the event you do not pass they will provide you with additional resources to help you pass the next time you take the exam. Some schools have agreements with various organizations. If your school does not have any formal affiliation, then be sure to be selective when choosing a program. Read their reviews and ask recent graduates who have successfully taken the NCLEX for advice.

Taking the licensure exam can be quite stressful so it is very helpful to employ strategies that will help decrease your stress and anxiety. You may employ simple breathing and relaxation techniques or learn how to meditate. You may also seek professional help if you feel you cannot address this issue on your own. Listening to music or engaging in activities can also be very helpful. There are many types of complementary alternative medicine that may be helpful in reducing stress and anxiety. Some examples are:

- Meditation
- Reiki
- Aromatherapy
- Hypnosis
- Deep breathing and relaxation
- Massage
- Therapeutic touch

Another great way to prepare for NCLEX and to study for your theory/clinical courses is to buy some NCLEX or licensure review books. Completing practice questions is quite helpful for learning content and learning how to prioritize and think critically. Rogers (2010) conducted a qualitative study on student success in an associate degree program and identified several themes such as good study habits, faculty support, and critical-thinking skills. "Students also expressed that completing practice questions and attending NCLEX-RN workshops and courses were instrumental to their success on the NCLEX-RN examination" (Rogers, 2010, p. 99).

It is a good idea to start practicing questions in your nursing fundamentals course and continue to do so in all of your courses. You can focus on content-specific questions that relate to your courses. After you graduate and are focused on preparing for your licensure exam you should complete all types of questions. Some students make a daily goal for themselves. For example, they might plan to complete 50 questions per day. If your school offers a predictor exam you can use those scores to develop a targeted plan of study. Even if your school does not offer a predictor exam you can complete a practice exam to identify your areas of weaknesses. Furthermore, after completing a vigorous nursing program you should be well aware of your strengths and weaknesses. Some students complete a focus review on their weak areas and just review practice questions on the content they have mastered.

FAILING THE LICENSURE EXAM

Our greatest glory is not in never failing, but in rising up every time we fail.

—Ralph Waldo Emerson

This quote by Ralph Waldo Emerson is right on target. Being able to bounce back from adversity is not easy but is something we must all learn how to do if we want to live life to the fullest. Everyone hopes to pass his or her licensure exam on the first try, unfortunately, not everyone is successful. In fact, according to Simon et al. (2013) the rate of failure for the NCLEX-RN is approximately 3,000 per year. Although it is very upsetting to fail it is important not to get discouraged. There are many reasons why a person does not do well on the first try and it does not mean that you will never realize your dream of becoming a registered professional nurse. Granted you may be filled with self-doubt and fearful to retake the exam, however, you must overcome this fear and develop a new plan and strategy for success. You will need to do some critical self-analysis to figure out what went wrong. Perhaps you were extremely anxious and could not focus on the questions. Or you took too long to respond to each question. Perhaps you needed to prepare more by reviewing concepts and completing more review questions. Maybe you didn't take a review class. Whatever the reason, you need to figure it out and make a new plan because you don't want to wait too long to retake the exam.

Another major factor in passing the licensure exam relates to potential language barriers. If English is not your primary language and you are taking the licensure exam in the United States it may be difficult to understand the intent of the questions based on the way they are worded. Furthermore, many academic institutions in other countries use essay questions rather than multiple choice on their exams (Hansen & Beaver, 2012). According to Olson (2012), "English as a second language (ESL) nursing students are a subpopulation of minority students who often struggle in nursing school and on licensure examinations" (p. 26). Students can be proficient in English but it may take 5 to 7 years for students to develop the more formal understanding required for college (Hansen & Beaver, 2012). "To improve their language skills, ESL students need to practice all four components of language proficiency: reading, listening, speaking, and writing" (Hansen & Beaver, 2012, p. 247). Joining a diverse study group, practicing multiple-choice questions, and completing reading comprehension exercises can be very helpful.

If you are an ELS student you should explore all the options available to you to help you to comprehend the complexities of the English language. On the other hand, if you are taking the exam in another country in a language other than English you will face the same challenges.

Remember, as Michael Chang says, "If at first you don't succeed, try, try, try, try, and try again."

In addition to passing your licensure exam there may be other requirements needed for licensure. For example, in New York all nurses and other health care providers must complete mandatory courses on child abuse and infection control. Although the child abuse course is only taken one time the infection control course must be taken every 4 years.

RENEWING YOUR LICENSE

All countries and states have policies and procedures for renewing one's license. This usually involves a fee and may require a personal statement that you have not been involved in any disciplinary or legal altercations. You may also be required to earn a certain amount of continuing-education credits when registering to renew your license. For example, in California nurses need to complete 30 hours of formal continuing-education credits every 2 years. Every state and country is different so it is best to review the guidelines for the state that you reside in or plan to practice in. You may hold licenses in different areas as long as you meet the requirements for the area. If you are licensed in a state within the United States and wish to work in another state you will be able to apply for reciprocity, which means you will not need to take another licensure exam. However, you will need to meet all the other requirements.

TOP 10 TIPS FOR RN LICENSURE SUCCESS

1. Begin preparing on your first day of nursing school.
2. Maintain a high GPA.
3. Read your textbooks.

4. Develop good study skills.

5. Join a study group.

6. Take a prep class.

7. Develop a formalized plan for success.

8. Complete a certain number of practice questions every day.

9. Engage in self-care and relaxation techniques.

10. Take advantage of all the resources that are available.

SUMMARY

This chapter focused on the NCLEX licensure exam. The significance of the exam was discussed as was the fact that all countries have licensure exams but will have different exams and procedures. Currently in the United States all states administer the same exam, which is developed by the National Council of State Boards of Nursing. Passing your licensure exam is the culmination of your educational journey; it gives you entry into professional practice. Unfortunately, not everyone is successful the first time he or she takes the licensure exam so it is important to develop a plan for success. There are many different strategies that one can employ and several of these were discussed in the chapter. Because everyone learns differently it is best to use a variety of strategies. If you are taking the licensure exam in the United States you will want to be familiar with Bloom's taxonomy as the questions have been developed based on the higher order questions of this taxonomy. You will also want to review the NLCEX test plan, which is available on the NCSBN's website and is updated every 3 years. If you are a nursing student in another country you will want to review your nursing board's website for information regarding the licensure exam. A brief discussion about failing the licensure exam was included in this chapter. Although no one wants to think about failing the licensure exam there is a possibility that it will happen so it is important to be prepared and have a plan for retaking the exam. Because study groups are extremely helpful for your courses and your licensure exam a template was provided to assist you when organizing your study group.

Discussion Questions

1. List three predictors of licensure success.
2. Discuss ways to prepare for the RN licensure exam.
3. Describe the key components of a study group.
4. What are the domains of Bloom's taxonomy?
5. What are some strategies you can use to reduce stress and anxiety?
6. What are the main categories included on the NCLEX-RN exam?
7. What strategies might be helpful to an ESL student?
8. What is the significance of the licensure exam?
9. In the Unites States how many people fail the NCLEX every year?
10. Where can you find information about the licensure exam for your state or country?

Suggested Learning Activities

- Develop a plan for preparing for your licensure exam.
- Identify at least three formal prep courses that you might take.
- Purchase or borrow at least one review book.
- Interview two nurses who have taken the licensure exam in the past year.
- Explore your board of nursing for information about the exam and licensing requirements for your state.

REFERENCES

Anderson, L. W. (1994). Research on teaching and teacher education. In L. W. Anderson & L. A. Sosniak (Eds.), *Bloom's taxonomy: A forty-year retrospective* (pp. 1–8). Chicago, IL: The University of Chicago Press.

ATI Testing. (2014). Retrieved from https://www.atitesting.com/

Aucoin, J., & Treas, L. (2005). Assumptions and realities of the NCLEX-RN. *Nursing Education Perspectives, 26*(5), 268–271.

Bloom, B. S., Engelhart, M. D., Furst, E. J., Hill, W. H., & Krathwohl, D. R. (Eds.). (1956). *Taxonomy of educational objectives: The classification of educational goals, handbook I— Cognitive domain.* New York: David McKay Company.

Bonis, S., Taft, L., & Wendler, M. (2007). Strategies to promote success on the NCLEX-RN: An evidence-based approach using the ACE Star Model of Knowledge Transformation. *Nursing Education Perspectives, 28*(2), 82–87.

Embassy of the United States Dublin, Ireland. (n.d.). *Nursing in the United States.* Retrieved from http://www.dublin.usembassy.gov/ireland/nursing.htm

Fischer, M., Boshoff, E., & Ehlers, V. (2001). Student nurses' needs for developing basic study skills. *Curationis, 24*(1), 66–73.

Hansen, E., & Beaver, S. (2012). Faculty support for ESL nursing students: Action plan for success. *Nursing Education Perspectives, 33*(4), 246–250.

Homard, C. M. (2013). Impact of a standardized test package on exit examination scores and NCLEX-RN outcomes. *Journal of Nursing Education, 52*(3), 175–178. doi: 10.3928/01484834-20130219-01

Lavandera, R., Whalen, D. M., Perkel, L. K., Hackett, V., Molnar, D., Steffey, C., & Harris, J. (2011). Value-added of HESI exam as a predictor of timely first-time RN licensure. *International Journal of Nursing Education Scholarship, 8*(1), 1–12. doi:10.2202/1548–923X.2152

Lavin, J., & Rosario-Sim, M. G. (2013). Understanding the NCLEX: How to increase success on the revised 2013 examination. *Nursing Education Perspectives, 34*(3), 196–198.

National Council of State Boards of Nursing. (2009). *NCLEX examination pass rates.* Retrieved from *https://www.ncsbn.org/1237.htm*

National Council of State Boards of Nursing. (2013). NCLEX-RN® examination test plan for the National Council Licensure Examination for Registered Nurses. Chicago. IL: Author. Retrieved from https://www.ncsbn.org/

Olson, M. (2012). English-as-a-second language (ESL) nursing student success: a critical review of the literature. *Journal of Cultural Diversity, 19*(1), 26–32.

Raman, J. (2013). Nursing student success in an associate degree program. *Teaching & Learning In Nursing, 8*(2), 50–58. doi:10.1016/j.teln.2012.12.001

Rogers, T. (2010). Prescription for success in an associate degree nursing program. *Journal of Nursing Education, 49*(2), 96–100. doi:10.3928/01484834-20091022-03

Romeo, E. M. (2013). The predictive ability of critical thinking, nursing GPA, and SAT scores on first-time NCLEX-RN performance. *Nursing Education Perspectives, 34*(4), 248–253.

Sewell, J., Culpa-Bondal, F., & Colvin, M. (2008). Nursing program assessment and evaluation: Evidence-based decision making improves outcomes. *Nurse Educator, 33*(3), 109–112.

Shelton, E. N. (2012). A model of nursing student retention. *International Journal of Nursing Education Scholarship, 9*(1), 1–16. doi:10.1515/1548-923X.2334

Simon, E. B., McGinniss, S. P., & Krauss, B. J. (2013). Predictor Variables for NCLEX-RN Readiness Exam Performance. *Nursing Education Perspectives, 34*(1), 18–24.

CHAPTER 8

Strategies for Securing Your First Position

The only person you are destined to become is the person you decide to be.

—Ralph Waldo Emerson

OBJECTIVES

After reading this chapter, the reader will be able to:

- Discuss strategies for securing one's first position
- Identify key components of a job search
- Develop a résumé and cover letter
- Understand the interview process
- Discuss key components of professional behavior
- Understand the relationship between personality testing and hiring

The road to becoming a registered professional nurse is somewhat long and winding, however, with each triumph you get closer to your goal. Once you pass your licensure exam, or are close to taking your exam, the next step is to secure a position. Consider for a moment Dorothy and her journey to Oz. Her path was filled with twists and turns and obstacles. However, she met friends and foes along the way. The friends helped her navigate her journey, similar to the mentors and role models who will help you on your path. Dorothy could have easily given up her dream of finding Oz and returning home because of the adversity she faced. However, she continued on her path and actually became

119

stronger along the way. She also learned that she was the one who had to solve her own problems and that indeed she had the power to do so but didn't realize it. Similar to Dorothy you will continue on your long and winding yellow brick road as you transition into professional practice. And although it would be nice to believe that the challenges will end after you secure your first position; this is not the case. Sure, you will have many rewards and positive experiences. However, your path will continue for many years and if you could see into the future you would be amazed at the incredible life-changing experiences you will have as a nurse. Not all experiences will be what you hoped or planned, however, they will all help to shape you as a person and a nurse.

Securing one's first nursing position can be very challenging, especially during times of economic downturn. Our world is constantly changing and some years there are job shortages, whereas others years there are nursing shortages (Buerhaus et al., 2007). Currently, we are in somewhat of a mixed environment. Due to the economic downturn and effects of globalization there has been a shift from full-time employment to contractual employment in Canada. However, with some improvements in the economy most new nurses are seeking more permanent full-time employment. In response to this a new program was implemented in Ontario by the government with funding available to health care organizations who participate in the program. This program is designed for new graduate nurses. According to Baumann et al. (2013), "In 2007, the MOHLTC [Ministry of Health and Long-Term Care] created the Nursing Graduate Guarantee (NGG). This health and human resource policy was designed to increase the availability of permanent full-time job opportunities for new graduate nurses" (p. 360). Although the employers who did participate in the program found it beneficial, only 20% of the 1,198 health care organizations participated (Baumann et al. 2013). One hopes more organizations in Canada and other countries will implement similar programs. "A survey by the National Student Nurses Association showed 36% of newly licensed registered nurses (RN) graduating in 2011 were not working as registered nurses 4 months after graduation" (Kurtz, 2013, para. 2). However, according to Buerhaus et al. (2013) the market for nurses is growing due in part to the Affordable Care Act, the expanding population of older adults, and the impending retirement of the current workforce. It is certainly more challenging for new graduates to secure their first position; however, this relates to geographic location, as some areas are still experiencing a nursing shortage. The good news is that there are strategies that you can use to assist in obtaining your first position. Similar to your licensure exam you also need to start preparing for your professional role on the first day of nursing school. Because the market is so competitive recruiters are highly selective and therefore you want to be a "shining star" and always conduct yourself in a professional manner. As discussed previously your grade point average (GPA) is related to licensure success, and it is also related to your success in obtaining your first position.

PROFESSIONAL ROLE

Transitioning from the student role to professional role is your next major hurdle. Although you have been preparing for this role throughout nursing school life is now very different because you are not under the collective wings of your faculty. Transitioning into professional practice can be very challenging and the literature is filled with statistics and facts about "reality shock," job dissatisfaction, and "new nurse turnover" (Almada et al., 2004; Beecroft et al., 2007; Dyess & Sherman, 2009). Challenges include increased accountability, role transition, higher acuity environment, and performance expectations (Trepenair et al., 2012). These issues will be discussed in greater detail throughout the rest of the book. On a more positive note many new graduates are offered positions in organizations that offer comprehensive orientation and ongoing support and they have a very positive transition. One of the major differences from student to new-graduate nurse is the autonomy and responsibility that come with your professional role. You will need to leave the nest, test your wings, and learn how to fly solo. Although you will be collaborating with other nurses and various members of the health care team, after your orientation you will need to complete your assessments, patient care, documentation, and interprofessional collaboration without the guidance or supervision of your faculty member or preceptor. This can be exciting and terrifying at the same time. It is helpful to remember you are not the only one to feel insecure as everyone feels somewhat overwhelmed when he or she transitions into the professional role. And for the most part you will have a support system available to you so be sure to let others know when you need support and guidance.

JOB SEARCH

There are multiple ways to search for a position, especially in this era of technology where almost anything can be located on the Internet. Most health care organizations have websites where they share information about available positions. Qualifications required and steps for applying are also included. Many organizations use an online system, whereas some require an e-mail, fax, or hardcopy submission. There are also trade magazines such as *ADVANCE for Nurses* and websites such as Spectrum.com that include informative articles, continuing education opportunities, and a classified section listing job opportunities. They also host career fairs both virtual and in person where you can meet directly with recruiters from various health care organizations. Networking and personal contacts are also a good source for information regarding available positions. A good place to begin is with the career counseling services at your college; however, not all colleges/universities offer this service. Another option is to explore opportunities at the various clinical sites you attended as a student. Many students make a great impression and develop professional relationships with the nurse managers, preceptors, and staff nurses on the units where they completed their clinical rotations. Professional organizations may also share information regarding available positions and members may be available to mentor you as your seek your first nursing position.

STRATEGIES FOR OBTAINING FIRST POSITION

When you begin your job search, the positions available for newly minted nurses may be abundant or quite scarce depending on the market and the economy. The current situation, although improved in some areas, is that although there are positions available many health care organizations are recruiting for experienced nurses and/or those with a BSN (bachelor of science in nursing). This presents a "catch-22" if you will; how do you obtain experience if no one is willing to hire you? Thankfully, there are still many organizations that will hire new-graduate nurses with an associate degree or a bachelor's degree, although many prefer the bachelor's degree. Furthermore, some hospitals will hire nurses with associate degrees if the nurse agrees to earn a bachelor's degree within 5 years. Because of the current demand for nurses who hold a baccalaureate degree, some states now have dual-degree programs in which a student can enroll in both an associate degree program and a bachelor's program. The student is eligible to take the licensure exam at the completion of the third year and may then work part time as the final year is completed.

Similar to your preparation for your licensure exam, preparation for your first nursing position should also begin on the day you enter the nursing program to improve your chances of being hired in an unpredictable marketplace. The job market is very competitive and recruiters are highly selective so you need to show them that you are serious about your professional role. Doing well in your courses is of the utmost importance as GPA is often considered, especially if you are applying for a summer externship, residency program, or fellowship. Conducting a brief search on the Internet reveals the GPA required for a summer externship ranges from 2.75 to 3.25. Prelicensure externships are a wonderful way to gain experience and prepare you for your future professional practice role. Externships are not mandatory and are not a formal part of your academic program (Cappel et al., 2013). The application process is competitive and the program usually runs over the summer break for 8 to 10 weeks, although there are shorter programs that may be offered during the winter break. These types of programs provide student nurses with theoretical concepts and clinical expertise. Students also develop professional relationships and are exposed to different clinical areas. During the externship you will be mentored by a nurse preceptor and there are theoretical and clinical concepts taught throughout the experience. Some prelicensure externships are paid positions, whereas others are unpaid. Whatever the case they provide invaluable experience and are also associated with future employment. Oftentimes, after you complete your summer externship you will be offered a per diem nursing assistant job where you can continue to gain experience and network with nurses and managers. The requirements vary based on the organization so you will need to do your homework and explore opportunities in your area. Furthermore, your school may have a career counseling officer who you can consult with about these types of opportunities. The ideal time to complete an externship is during the summer before your senior year and applications are usually due in February or March. You will also need to submit a résumé and cover letter, in addition to letters of recommendation, so you need to give adequate time for soliciting your recommendation from one of two of your professors. It is a good idea to include one from your clinical instructor and one from your theory professor. In this age of technology most organizations have an online application and processes for submitting the other items. Of course, they will require an official transcript so you will need to order this from your school. The application process, whether for an externship, internship, residency, or staff nurse position, is very similar, and requires meticulous attention to detail.

The benefits of networking cannot be stressed enough. According to Owens and Young (2008), networking is one of the most effective ways to connect and is especially helpful in connecting job seekers with future employers. Networking is the development of business relationships via the sharing of information among interested individuals or organizations. As a nursing student you will have many opportunities to network and so it is important to develop positive relationships with your peers, faculty, and preceptors. It is especially important to network in all of your clinical sites as these connections will be most beneficial when you are ready to apply for a position.

When networking, Owens and Young (2008) suggest the following:

- Listen and be polite
- Do not expect anything
- Be dependable and reliable
- Remember to say "thank you"

These guidelines are very important and you always want to be professional in all of your communications whether in person, via e-mail, or on social media. Networking can be difficult if you are introverted or shy. This is something you will have to work on because your role as a nurse will require you to communicate with many different people. You may want to role-play with your friends, or seek assistance from your faculty or counselor.

A mentor is also vitally important and one should plan on having one or two mentors throughout her or his nursing career. A mentor can often guide you and help you in your search for a new position. The role of mentors and the relationship one forms with his or her mentors will be more fully discussed in Chapter 10.

Developing a well-written exemplary résumé and cover letter are vitally important in securing a position (see Appendix). Portfolios are also very helpful when applying for a professional position (see Chapter 6). Initially you will submit your résumé and cover letter, most often in an electronic format. If you are called for an interview, then you can bring a hard copy of your portfolio or inquire with the recruiter if they would like to review your portfolio. Your résumé and cover letter are a reflection of you and will be the deciding factors in whether or not you are called in for an interview. Poorly written documents with errors will go into the slush pile. You certainly don't want that to happen so be sure to have someone critique your documents prior to submitting them. Be sure to check what services are available at your college because many of them offer consultation with experts who will help you prepare your résumé, cover letter, and review interview skills via role-play and mock interviews.

Professional organizations offer many benefits—continuing education, journals, and certification review courses. There are many to choose from and nurses usually join the organizations that relate to their specialty, for example, the American Association of Critical Care Nursing, or the Academy of Medical–Surgical Nurses, American Nurses Association, just to name a few. Joining a professional organization is a great way to network and many of them offer reduced rates for students. Some of them have annual conferences where you can network with nurses from many different locations. As a student you should join the National Student Nurses Association, which offers students many benefits and student leadership opportunities. Some schools provide automatic membership for all their students in the National Student Nurses Association so be sure to inquire with your school and make some time to get involved.

Volunteerism is another wonderful way to network and gain access into a health care organization. Although you may not be functioning in a clinical capacity you will be in a hospital environment and can work on your communication skills with patients, families, and a variety of health care professionals. You will have many opportunities to network and can learn more about specific units within the hospital system. This will also look wonderful on your résumé and demonstrate your commitment to your profession.

An internship or residency is highly desirable and beneficial, and according to many experts should be available to all new graduates. According to Capel et al. (2013) the nurse model for the nurse residency program was based on the work of Patricia Benner (1984). Although the programs may vary, a standardized curriculum includes a focus on communication, patient-centered care, organizational skills, and leadership. Cappel et al. (2013) state that, "Graduate nurses should seek out organizations that offer nurse residency programs (NRPs) to foster their professional development" (p. 27).

Internships and residency programs are often available to new graduate nurses who have passed their licensure exam. Unfortunately, there are not enough programs to accommodate all the new graduates and the programs are very competitive. If you follow the advice in this chapter you will greatly increase your chances of being selected into one of these prestigious programs. Internships, residencies, and fellowships are offered to new graduate nurses most often with the stipulation that they first must pass the licensure exam. These programs provide from 6 months to 1 year of orientation, continuing education, precepting, and mentoring. Oftentimes they are for specialty areas such as critical care or the operating room. The Institute of Medicine's Report *The Future of Nursing* supports and recommends a transition-to-practice residency program for all new nurses and advanced practice nurses (Robert Wood Johnson Foundation, 2010). Most experts agree that a residency program is warranted, but unfortunately there are not enough funds to support this goal, or at least that is the perception because some studies have demonstrated the cost-effectiveness of nurse residency programs. For example, Trepanier et al. (2012) posit that based on their study nurse residency programs should be viewed as an "investment instead of an expense" (p. 214). Taylor Keasler, a new-graduate nurse, found her residency program to be invaluable. It was a year long and included formal classes, precepting, and mentoring. She states that retention rates of new graduates at her hospital went from 71.1 % in 2007 to 89.7% in 2011 after the implementation of the nurse residency program (Keasler, 2013). The benefits of nurse residency programs include improved retention rates, cost benefits, successful transition of the new nurse, job satisfaction, and quality of care (Cappel et al., 2013; Trepanier et al., 2012).

The process for residency application is complex and will require you to complete and submit a variety of documents. Each organization has different requirements so be sure to check the websites of all organizations to which you are submitting an application. You can expect to submit the following documents:

- Application
- Cover letter (see sample in Appendix)
- Résumé (see sample in Appendix)
- Detailed list of clinical rotations
- Essay (topic may be provided)
- Official transcript (must be ordered via school)
- Portfolio
- Letters of recommendation

This is an important application so be sure to check and double check all of your documents. You do not want to lose out on an opportunity because of careless mistakes. Be sure to have someone review your résumé, cover letter, and essay. If you are submitting to more than one hospital be sure to tailor your documents to the specific organization and follow their guidelines exactly as stated. For example, if an essay is required and has a suggested topic and word count you must adhere to this guideline. Some organizations will not even consider applications that do not meet the exact guidelines. You will also want to be prepared for a potential interview.

APPLICATION PROCESS

The application process involves the development of a well-written résumé and cover letter (see examples), in addition to completion of an application. Many organizations now use an electronic system for completing an online application and submitting required documentation.

This may require a Word document or a pdf or some other version. Prior to starting your online application you should have a high-quality polished résumé and cover letter to submit. If possible have a faculty member or career counselor review your résumé and cover letter. The key is to be concise and only include important items. Recruiters read hundreds of résumés and do not have time to read lengthy or wordy documents. You also want to be sure you are qualified for the position before you spend time completing the application.

The cover letter (see template) is vitally important as it is your introduction and the first impression you will make on recruiters. The cover letter should be designed in a way that demonstrates that you are the perfect candidate for the position (Donahue, 1997). The cover letter is a one-page document that is written in professional language. It should be tailored to the specific organization and position you are applying for. Begin with an introduction and brief overview of your background, then identify the position you are applying for. In the next paragraph you should detail why you are qualified for this position (Hunt, 2013). The final paragraph should show your enthusiasm for the position (Donahue, 1997). There should be great attention to detail with emphasis on spelling and grammar. Each cover letter should be specific to the position. Also, be sure to find out the name of the recruiter so that you can personalize your letter.

The résumé is part and parcel with the cover letter and requires careful development and concise statements. Many experts recommend that the résumé be one page long, so you need to communicate all the vital information in as few words as possible. Résumés should "paint a picture of your skills and experience" (Becze, 2008, p. 29). You should use action words and use present tense for your current position and past tense for previous positions. The font should be 12-point black Times New Roman on quality bond white or ivory paper (Cardillo, 2001). You may use bullet points and appropriate spacing when listing detailed information about a position to ensure readability (Becze, 2008). "The goal of an effective résumé is to present your competencies and credentials in an inviting way. Résumés that attract the attention of employers introduce an interesting candidate who appears to have "what it takes" to step into a job immediately" (Donahue, 1997, p. 1). There is no right or wrong way to develop your résumé, however, according to Shakoor (2001), the most common and preferred format is the chronological format (see template), which lists education and experience in chronological order. The other option is the functional format, which lists skills or competencies (Hunt, 2013). Because the résumé and cover letter are so important you may want to consult with a professional service to assist you in their development. There are also many resources available online and templates that may be available on your computer. Even after you have secured your position it is important to keep your résumé updated and current because you will need it for future positions and when you are returning to school for your advanced degree.

INTERVIEW PROCESS

The interview process can be a daunting experience and, similar to other experiences, the first one is the hardest. The key to a successful interview is to be prepared and professional. Be sure to arrive early, be courteous, shake hands, allow the interviewer to speak without interruption, and thank everyone at the end of the interview. Make sure you have all the required documents and other information with you such as dates of employment, names of your direct supervisor, and his or her contact information. You should also follow-up with a thank-you note either by e-mail or snail mail (Ratliff, 2010). You definitely should be knowledgeable about the organization—the philosophy, type of unit, patient population, and orientation program are all important. Most organizations have websites where you can locate all the vital information you require. You should also be prepared to share your strengths and weaknesses. Performance-based interviews are often conducted in nursing so you need to be prepared to answer situational questions that involve different clinical scenarios. Try to respond with examples that demonstrate your knowledge, caring, passion, and professionalism. Although you should be able to answer these types of questions without looking at your notes you may want to have a notebook handy for when it is your turn to ask some questions (Hawke, 2003). You should also explore whether a simulation scenario will be a part of the interview process as many organizations are now including this as part of the interview. With luck, you will be exposed to simulation while you are a student so that you will be comfortable with this type of experience.

You may go through a series of interviews or just have one with the recruiter. Or you may be asked to perform an assessment or give an example of a shift-to-shift report. As mentioned, some organizations use simulation and may ask you to demonstrate a focused assessment. Recruiters realize you may be nervous and will allow for that, nevertheless they do expect you to be prepared. Therefore, you need to do your homework, seek expert help, and participate in mock interviews. Develop a list of potential questions and responses that might be posed to you during the interview. You should also develop a list of questions you would like to ask the recruiter/interviewer. For example, you might ask about orientation, precepting, or professional development programs. Most experts caution against discussing salary on the initial interview. Try to allow the recruiter to speak without interrupting and be careful not to share too much personal information. It is best to focus on the professional aspects of the interview. You may also want to do some deep breathing and relaxation exercises prior to your interview. You should also be prepared to be interviewed by the nurse manager or quite possibly the staff nurses. If you are prepared you should be fine, no one expects you to be perfect, especially as a new graduate.

Personality Testing and the Interview Process

The interview process is highly varied based on organization and type of position. Some organizations use personality testing in their interviews. There are certainly pros and cons to this type of testing and there is no real consensus on their efficacy (Scroggins et al., 2009). Organizations do not usually share with the candidates the type of interview they will be conducting so it is a good idea to be prepared for as many scenarios as possible. One of the common personality tests used during interviews is the General Mental Ability (GMA) Test.

"People with demonstrated high levels of GMA seem to acquire job knowledge with greater speed and depth, and this boosts job performance" (Scroggins et al., 2009, p. 68). Certainly, organizations want to hire candidates with the greatest potential especially as it is very expensive to hire and train a new employee. Personality or behavioral interviews have no right or wrong responses and therefore you should not let this cause you undue stress and anxiety. You may not even be aware that the interview is based on the GMA, and you should answer questions to the best of your ability. You may want to consult with other recent graduates who have gone through the interview process as they can provide you with some helpful tips and advice.

PROFESSIONALISM

"Professionalism" is an all-encompassing term for all the behaviors and actions that you perform as a professional nurse. When one enters nursing school he or she embarks on a path to professionalism. Developing one's professional identity is required of all professions; however, nursing has faced many challenges in this area (Deppoliti, 2008). Nurses must do what they can to improve their public image and play a more influential role in health care by increasing their visibility and engaging in public discourse on the vital issues that impact health and wellness (Hoeve et al., 2014). "Nursing graduates should be knowledgeable, competent and professional. These qualities will be reflected in the practice of skilled practitioners who are able to make sound clinical judgments resulting in quality patient care" (Williams & Day, 2009, p.1). Student nurses are exposed to various aspects of professionalism throughout their nursing programs. Mentors, role models, and peers can help students to understand the importance of professional behavior. Development of this behavior "encompasses values and norms, as well as skills and behaviors" (Secrest et al., 2003, p. 78). Secrest et al. (2003) posit that three themes of professionalism in new nurses emerged in their qualitative study: belonging, knowing, and affirmation. Clearly, new nurses need significant support and positive reinforcement and exemplary role models to guide them in their transition and continued development of professional behavior.

Communication is extremely important and we need to be cognizant of our written, verbal, and nonverbal communication. We need to be able to speak clearly and articulate our words in an intelligent and clear manner. Written communication must be exemplary. Whether writing a formal paper, letter, essay, or nursing notes we need to use proper grammar, spelling, and sentence structure. Our thoughts should be organized and make sense. Nonverbal communication should match our verbal communication. We must also be sensitive to cultural influences in regard to communication and professionalism. Having business cards for networking is very important and they can easily be created and printed on your home computer and printer.

The way we portray ourselves and our attire are other significant factors. There is an old adage, "dress for success," and this should be your mantra. When preparing for interviews you want to dress neatly and conservatively. A blue or black tailored skirt or pants suit are recommended. Hair should be styled or pulled back with jewelry at a minimum. You should have a briefcase to carry your important documents. Shoes should have medium heels and stockings should be neutral. You should not chew gum and your cellphone should be turned off or placed on vibrate and kept in your bag. Punctuality is very important so give yourself plenty of time to reach your location and find parking. Smiling is also helpful as you will portray a caring demeanor. Be careful not to use jargon or gestures that might be misconstrued.

Once you are hired into a position you will be required to dress in a certain way. As a new-graduate nurse you will most likely be required to wear a uniform. Many hospitals have adapted a standardized scrub top and bottom so you will need to find that out prior to beginning your new position. If you do not have a specific guideline regarding your attire, then you should opt for something conservative. Whether you wear a uniform or business attire you must always look professional. Clothing should be clean, pressed, and conservative. Uniforms should also be clean and pressed and in compliance with the dress code of your organization. Jewelry and other accessories should be basic and in compliance with dress codes. Many organizations prohibit nail polish or artificial nails due to issues with infection control. Similarly, hair should be pulled back so as not to compromise infection control or compromise the sterile field. Although some rules regarding dress code may seem irrelevant they do serve a purpose—portraying a professional image and decreasing incidence of cross-contamination. Several studies have been conducted on the relationship of professional attire and positive nursing image. "Researchers in a study of adult participants found that a white nurse's uniform conveyed the traits of confidence, reliability, competence, professionalism, and efficiency, and a uniform with a small print pattern conveyed traits of caring, attentiveness, cooperation, empathy, and being approachable" (Girard, 2009, p. 419). The starched white uniform and cap may be a thing of the past; nonetheless, exhibiting a professional image is critical for your own personal identity and as a representative of the nursing profession.

LETTERS OF RECOMMENDATION

Letters of recommendation and/or reference letters are required by most organizations. These letters are usually written by one of your faculty members or employers. Some organizations will stipulate the type of letter they require. You must be cognizant of the fact that everyone has a busy schedule and developing these letters takes time and attention on the part of the recommender. You should not list someone as a reference unless you have received permission from them. Therefore, you need to begin this process early, when you are preparing for your job search. Clinical faculty can be the perfect people to provide you with a recommendation; however, because many of them are adjuncts you need to make this request during the semester. As stated previously, some academic institutions have career counseling services that will maintain an individual file with your résumé, portfolio, and reference letters. Therefore, you can request these letters throughout your program. Remember, it is your responsibility to invite your recommender and to share the process with him or her, for example, the format of the letter and the process for submitting their letter. You should also send this person a copy of your résumé and accomplishments so he or she can personalize your letter. Some organizations have a standardized online format for reference letters so your recommender must be comfortable with technology and using an online submission service. You should consider this when you invite someone to write a letter of reference/ recommendation. You will need at least two individuals to recommend you. Try to select individuals who will be able to write a strong letter of support within the required deadline.

Top 10 Tips for Your Job Search

1. Maintain a high GPA.
2. Apply for a student externship.
3. Consult with a career counseling service if available.
4. Network and consult with your mentor.
5. Develop a well-written up-to-date résumé and cover letter.
6. Attend a career fair.
7. Join a professional organization.
8. Prepare for your interview by identifying your strengths and weaknesses.
9. Participate in mock interviews.
10. Research all the organizations you are applying to.

Summary

This chapter focused on strategies for securing one's first position as a new-graduate nurse. It included vital information on the professional role and strategies for securing one's first position. The importance of being prepared and professional was highlighted throughout the chapter. Vital information on the résumé, cover letter, and interview process was included, in addition to other key components related to strengthening yourself as an exemplary candidate in a competitive job market.

DISCUSSION QUESTIONS

1. Describe the difference between the student role and professional role.
2. List and discuss three strategies that you can use as a student that will make you more marketable.
3. What is the difference between a chronological and functional résumé?
4. What is the average length of a résumé?
5. What is the purpose of the cover letter?
6. Identify at least three sources for locating information about available positions.
7. Discuss ways to prepare for an interview.
8. What are three of your strengths in relation to your nursing role?
9. What are three of your weaknesses in relation to your nursing role?
10. Give five examples of professional behavior.

SUGGESTED LEARNING ACTIVITIES

- Develop a résumé and cover letter.
- Participate in mock interviews.
- Explore opportunities for externships, internships, and residency programs.
- Attend a career fair.

- Choose three health care organizations and review their process for submitting an application.
- Select one of the three organizations above and explore its website for information about the organization (e.g., mission, type of organization, inpatient beds, nursing philosophy, etc.)

APPENDIX

SAMPLE COVER LETTER

Ms. Helen Gray, MS, RN
Nurse Recruiter
General Hospital
2395 Golden Sun Street
Somerset, NY 23876

Date

Dear Ms. Gray,

I would like to apply for the nurse residency position at....... (name of organization) My qualifications for this position are.............................. (include relevant experience).

Thank-you for considering this application and I look forward to meeting with you at your earliest convenience.

Sincerely,

Judith Tenety

SAMPLE RÉSUMÉ

Marybeth Stevens
1214 Sunset Trail
Somerset, NY 10987
654-987-4312
mstevens@olamail.com

Education

New Jersey College, Silver Springs, NJ Bachelor of Science in Nursing	5/2013
Somerset County High School Diploma	6/2009

Professional Experience

General Hospital, Somerset, NJ   9/12–present

Nursing Assistant
- Provide patient care for 8 patients under the supervision of a registered nurse
- Conduct patient safety rounds

Nurse Externship—Critical Care   6/12–9/12

Clinical Rotations

NJ Memorial Hospital Center, Somerset, NJ   Nursing Leadership
Somerset Medical Center, Somerset, NJ   Medical/Surgical Nursing
New Jersey Presbyterian Hospital, Newark, NJ   Psychiatric Mental Health
Somerset Children's Hospital, Somerset, NJ   Pediatric Nursing
Montefiore North Division Hospital, Bronx, NY   Maternal/Newborn Nursing
New Jersey Presbyterian Hospital, Newark, NJ   Medical/Surgical Nursing

Volunteer

General Hospital   2010–2012

Certifications

- Basic Cardiac Life Support (BCLS)

Honors/Awards

- Student Nurse Award—General Hospital

Professional Organizations

- National Student Nurse Association
- American Association of Critical Care Nurses

REFERENCES

Almada, P., Carafoli, K., Flattery, J. B., French, D. A., & McNamara, M. (2004). Improving the retention rate of newly graduated nurses. *Journal for Nurses in Staff Development, 20*(6), 268–273.

Baumann, A., Hunsberger, M., & Crea-Arsenio, M. (2013). Full-time work for nurses: Employers' perspectives. *Journal of Nursing Management, 21*(2), 359–367. doi:10.1111/j.1365-2834.2012.01391.x

Becze, E. (2008). Staying on top: Resume writing, part 1—Develop a self-inventory. *ONS Connect, 23*(2), 29.

Beecroft, P., Dorey. F., & Wenten, M. (2007). Turnover intention in new graduate nurses: A multivariate analysis. *Journal of Advanced Nursing, 62*, 41–52.

Benner, P. E. (1984). *From novice to expert: Excellence and power in clinical nursing practice.* Meulo Park, CA: Addison-Wesley

Buerhaus, P., Auerbach, D., & Staiger, D. (2007). Recent trends in the registered nurse labor market in the U.S.: Short-run swings on top of long-term trends. *Nursing Economic$, 25*(2), 59–67.

Buerhaus, P., Auerbach, D., Staiger, D., & Muench, U. (2013). Projections of the long-term growth of the registered nurse workforce: A regional analysis. *Nursing Economic$, 31*(1), 13–17.

Cappel, C. A., Hoak, P. L., & Karo, P. A. (2013). Nurse residency programs: What nurses need to know. *Pennsylvania Nurse, 68*(4), 22–28.

Cardillo, D. (2001). Career path. Résumé writing: Make a good impression. *Nursing, 31*(3), 77–79.

Deppoliti, D. (2008). Exploring how new registered nurses construct professional identity in hospital settings. *Journal of Continuing Education in Nursing, 39*(6), 255–262. doi:10.3928/00220124-20080601-03

Donahue, D. (1997). Career corner. Your résumé and cover letter. *Massachusetts Nurse, 67*(8), 3.

Dyess, S., & Sherman, R. (2009). The first year of practice: New graduate nurses' transition and learning needs. *Journal of Continuing Education in Nursing. 40*(9), 403–410.

Girard, N. (2011). Perception of nurse professionalism based on the uniform. *AORN Journal, 94*(4), 419–420. doi:10.1016/j.aorn.2011.07.004

Hawke, M. (2003). *Ten killer interview tips.* Retrieved from https://www.Nurse.com

Hoeve, Y., Jansen, G., & Roodbol, P. (2014). The nursing profession: Public image, self-concept and professional identity. A discussion paper. *Journal of Advanced Nursing, 70*(2), 295–309. doi:10.1111/jan.12177

Hunt, D. (2013). *The new nurse educator: Mastering academe.* New York: Springer Publishing.

Keasler, T. (2013). Nurse residency program empowers new grads. *American Nurse, 45*(4), 13.

Kurtz, A. (2013, January 14). For nursing jobs, new grads need not apply. *CNN Money.* Retrieved from http://money.cnn.com/2013/01/14/news/economy/nursing-jobs-new-grads/

Owens, L., & Young, P. (2008). You're hired! The power of networking. *Journal of Vocational Rehabilitation, 29*(1), 23–28.

Ratliff, P. (2010). *Interview tips for the job-seeking nurse.* Retrieved from https://www.Nurse.com

Robert Wood Johnson Foundation. (2010). *Initiative on the future of nursing.* Retrieved from https://www.thefutureofnursing.org

Scroggins, W., Thomas, S., & Morris, J. (2009). Psychological testing in personnel selection, Part III: The resurgence of personality testing. *Public Personnel Management, 38*(1), 67–77.

Secrest, J., Norwood, B., & Keatley, V. (2003). "I was actually a nurse": The meaning of professionalism for baccalaureate nursing students. *Journal of Nursing Education, 42*(2), 77–82.

Shakoor, T. (2001). Developing a professional résumé and cover letter that work. *Black Collegian, 32*(1), 16. Retrieved from http://www.blackcollegian.com/developing-a-professional-resume-and-cover-letter-that-work

Trepanier, S., Early, S., Ulrich, B., & Cherry, B. (2012). New graduate nurse residency program: A cost-benefit analysis based on turnover and contract labor usage. *Nursing Economic$, 30*(4), 207–214.

Williams, B., & Day, R. (2009). Employer perceptions of knowledge, competency, and professionalism of baccalaureate nursing graduates from a problem-based program. *International Journal of Nursing Education Scholarship, 6*(1), 1–11. doi:10.2202/1548-923X.1646

PART III

Transition Into Professional Practice

CHAPTER 9

Role of the Graduate Nurse

You have brains in your head. You have feet in your shoes. You can steer yourself in any direction you choose. You're on your own, and you know what you know. And you are the guy who'll decide where to go.

—Dr. Seuss

OBJECTIVES

After reading this chapter, the reader will be able to:

- Discuss the role expectations for the nurse generalist
- Identify key theoretical frameworks that inform transition of the new nurse
- Discuss the stages identified by Benner from novice to expert
- Understand work culture and group dynamics
- Understand the importance of liability insurance
- Describe additional certifications and courses required for ongoing role development

Students who complete a diploma program in nursing, an associate degree program in nursing, or a bachelor's degree program in nursing are prepared to sit for the licensure exam and to assume the role of nurse generalist. These programs share the common core nursing curriculum; however, the baccalaureate program includes a strong liberal arts foundation and additional courses that focus on critical-thinking skills, communication, and language. "Baccalaureate nursing programs encompass all of the course work taught in associate degree and diploma programs plus a more in-depth treatment of the physical and social sciences, nursing research, public and community health, nursing management, and the humanities" (AACN, 2014, para 4). According to the American Association of Colleges of Nurses (AACN, 2008) the role of the baccalaureate nurse generalist is derived from the discipline of nursing practice and includes being a provider of care, being a member of the profession, and being a manager of care.

According to the AACN (2008) the baccalaureate nurse generalist is prepared to:

- Work in a variety of settings
- Critically think and reason
- Provide holistic care across the life span
- Practice self-care
- Be a lifelong learner

These concepts create the very fabric of your development as a nurse and you will continue to develop and expand your knowledge and skills while transitioning into your professional practice role. As a newly minted baccalaureate nurse you will be expected to demonstrate your knowledge of these concepts.

According to the National League for Nursing (NLN; 2013) the following competencies must be achieved by the associate degree nurse:

- Human flourishing
- Nursing judgment
- Professional identity
- Spirit of inquiry

Human flourishing relates to advocacy for patients and families. Nursing judgment requires the associate degree nurse to provide safe quality care that is based on evidence and the integration of nursing science to promote health of patients within the family and community. Professional identity relates to integrity and ethical practices in one's role and a commitment to providing safe quality care and serving as an advocate for diverse patients. Nurses are expected to be committed to caring, evidenced-based practice, safety, quality care, and advocacy. Spirit of inquiry requires the nurse to use the evidence to offer new insights into the provision of quality care for patients, families, and communities (NLN, 2013).

Whether you have graduated from a diploma program, associate degree program, or baccalaureate program, as a new nurse you will be expected to serve as a nurse generalist and will continue to learn and develop as you transition from a student to new-graduate nurse. Your role will be somewhat similar to that which you experienced as a nursing student during your clinical rotation, although you will now be expected to work independently and demonstrate competency in all areas. When you first begin your new position you will be given a formal orientation and will most likely be precepted by an experienced nurse. This is an exciting time during which you will be totally immersed in your new role. The orientation program and strategies for a successful transition will be discussed in the next chapter. As a nurse generalist you are prepared to use the nursing process when providing safe quality care to patients, families, and communities in accordance with the Nurse Practice Act and informed by the American Nurses Association Code of Ethics.

Below is the Nurse Practice Act from New York state. Each state has an individualized Nurse Practice Act that is similar to this.

§6902. Definition of practice of nursing.

The practice of the profession of nursing as a registered professional nurse is defined as diagnosing and treating human responses to actual or potential health problems through such services as case finding, health teaching, health counseling, and provision of care supportive to or restorative of life and well-being, and executing medical regimens prescribed by a licensed physician, dentist or other licensed health care provider legally authorized under this title and in accordance with the commissioner's regulations. A nursing regimen shall be consistent with and shall not vary any existing medical regimen. (New York State Education Department [NYSED. gov], 2010)

This definition applies to all licensed professional nurses regardless of their educational preparation. As previously discussed it is vitally important to know and follow your state or country's Nurse Practice Act.

THEORETICAL FRAMEWORKS AND MODELS

Theoretical frameworks enlighten us to some of the stages and processes new employees may experience. One can be filled with self-doubt during this transition period, thinking he or she is alone and must be doing something wrong. However, this is not the case as everyone goes through a period of adjustment, with trials and tribulations and joys and successes. Admittedly each individual has a unique experience and therefore should not be overly concerned if his or her experience is different from their peers.

One well-known model that was developed by Dalton, Thompson, and Price (1977) outlines four stages that an individual experiences throughout his or her professional career. However, each stage may not be achieved. The four stages are *apprentice, colleague, mentor, and sponsor*. Each of these stages is unique and has distinct characteristics and needs such as mentoring, education, and support. Based on this framework, as a new nurse you would be considered an apprentice during your orientation period. When you are able to work independently and manage a complete assignment you would be considered a colleague. When you are at the stage in your development during which you become a preceptor you would be at the mentor stage.

Tyrell-Smith (2011) described the four stages of a successful career. The first stage is *training and development*, during which the new employee is oriented to the organization and the role. The second stage is *success*, which occurs when you reach a milestone, for example, the completion of your residency program in nursing. The third stage is *significance*, which relates to the impact you have on others in relation to the work that you do. *Continuation* is the fourth stage and relates to your continual development and influence. These stages were written from a business perspective but they can certainly relate to any career.

Some theories explain or predict challenges and issues faced by new nurses as they transition into their professional practice role. Kramer (1974) described *reality shock*, the conflict between role expectations of the new nurse and the reality that many new nurses experience (Kramer, 1974). Kramer (1974) described the phases a new nurse experiences as he or she transitions into professional practice as the honeymoon phase, the shock (rejection) phase, the recovery phase, and the resolution phase. During the *honeymoon phase* the new nurse views everything as wonderful and is excited about his or her new role. The *shock and rejection phase* occurs when the new nurse begins to experience conflict between what he or she was taught in school and what occurs in the real world. In this phase the new nurse may begin to experience signs of burnout, such as fatigue, anxiety, depression, and anger. In the *recovery phase* the nurse begins to look at things more objectively and tension and anxiety decrease. The *resolution phase* may end either positively or negatively. The nurse may learn to cope or he or she may leave nursing, or stay and experience burnout.

TRANSITION THEORY

Duchscher (2008) described a theory of successful transition in which new nurses embark on a journey and must go through the stages of *doing, being, and knowing*. In the *doing* stage the new nurse is involved in learning, performing, concealing, adjusting, and accommodating. If this phase is negative, the nurse would experience shock. The *being* stage involves searching, examining, doubting, questioning, and revealing. This stage may be positive or result in the nurse experiencing a crisis. The *knowing* stage involves separating, recovering, exploring, critiquing, and accepting. Duchscher (2008) posits the transition process usually takes 12 months; but the stages are not linear in nature. Inherent in a successful process is the presence of a structured orientation and mentoring programs. Duchscher (2009) has spent the past 10 years researching new-nurse transition and has developed a model of *transition shock* based on her findings. "Transition shock emerged as the experience of moving from the known role of a student to the relatively less familiar role of professionally practicing nurse" (Duchscher, 2009, p. 1105). When students transition into their practice role they expect that it will be similar to their experience as a student, however, this is often not the case. The model of transition shock developed by Duchscher (2009) includes the central tenets of knowledge, roles, responsibilities, and relationships with the mediators of loss, disorientation, doubt, and confusion, which have an effect on physical, intellectual, emotional, and social development. This theory applies to the initial 3 to 4 months of new-graduate nurse transition, when the new nurse engages in a process of adjustment that is motivated by responsibilities and relationships and involves sociocultural, intellectual, and developmental changes (Duchscher, 2009).

Duchscher (2009) suggests that educational institutions and industry collaborate on developing transition programs based on the issues identified in the transition shock model. Numerous studies have identified the challenges of transition and the strategies that can be employed to assist the new nurse with this process; this will be further discussed in the next chapter.

TRANSITIONS

Meleis (2007) described transition in regard to nurses who are dealing with patients who are experiencing a transition. "*Transition* denotes a change in health status, or in role relationships, expectations, or abilities"

(Meleis, 2007, p. 470). Coping and adapting are concepts that apply to transition. Nurses can help their patients learn coping skills and help them adapt to a change in physical or psychological domains. For example, a patient who has rheumatoid arthritis can be taught the importance of exercise, stress reduction, and healthy eating to deal with the physical and psychological effects of this disease. Each person is unique and therefore nurses must individualize their plan of care based on the specific needs of their patients. "Transition requires the person to incorporate new knowledge, to alter behavior, and therefore to change the definition of self in social context" (Meleis, 2007, p. 470). The transition process can be healthy, with the individual restructuring life routines and developing skills and knowledge. On the other hand the transition process can be unhealthy, with the individual maintaining unrealistic expectations or refusing opportunities to grow. Although Meleis (2007) did not write specifically about new-nurse transition one can easily see how this theory is applicable to new nurses. Furthermore, nurse researchers have used Meleis's (2007) theory to guide their research on nurse transition. For example, Flinter (2011) described the study she completed in 2010 on transition of nurse practitioners (NP) who completed a year-long residency program. The participants who completed the NP residency program had a successful transition and were able to overcome the challenges they faced. This study, although small, lends further support to the value of residency programs.

In summary, models and theories have been developed to explain the transition process and its negative and positive outcomes. All new graduates face challenges as they transition into their professional practice role. Understanding the transition process and its implications can help to lessen feelings of isolation and self-doubt. It is also vital that nurse managers, preceptors, and mentors understand this process so they can help new-graduate nurses develop coping and adaptation skills required for a smooth transition. Furthermore, all nurses must understand the role they play in the transition process in relation to their patients and families so they can help patients to develop coping and adaptation skills for the inevitable changes that come with illness.

NOVICE TO EXPERT: PATRICIA BENNER

The book *Novice to Expert* by Patricia Benner (1984) should be required reading for all student nurses as it helps the student to understand the growth and development he or she will experience as a student and when he or she transitions into professional practice and continues his or her journey. Benner (1984) based her model on the Dreyfus model, and described the stages that the nurse advances through from the novice to the expert. Although these stages are linear in nature there is no set pattern. Furthermore, one can be an expert as a critical care nurse, but, if he or she transitions to a new role (for example, as a psychiatric nurse), he or she will begin at the novice stage again. Understanding these stages can be comforting because we are often very self-critical and also have a tendency to compare ourselves with others. This can be very damaging as transition and development are done on an individual basis, and whether you are a fast learner or a slow learner advancing from one stage to the other takes commitment, support, time, and experience.

Benner (1984) described five stages of knowledge development—theoretical, practical, and clinical in relation to nurses when they transition into practice, or into a new type of practice or setting. The stages of development begin with the novice stage and culminate with the expert stage. The novice applies to nursing students when they first enter the clinical area and have little understanding of how the theoretical concepts relate to the clinical care of their patients. Nurses who enter a new clinical setting where they have limited experience are also considered to be novices. Novice nurses require support, mentoring, and encouragement, and can only function independently when very basic care is required. The second stage is advanced beginner, "who can demonstrate marginally acceptable performance" (Benner, 1984, p. 22). At this point the new nurse can "formulate principles that dictate actions in terms of both attributes and aspects" (Benner 1984, p. 23). The advanced beginner now has a frame of reference of important concepts and can apply them in the clinical setting, although with support and help in prioritizing care. The competence stage is reached after the nurse spends 2 to 3 years on a particular unit experiencing similar situations. At this stage the nurse can analyze and contemplate a problem and develop a plan of action. However, according to Benner (1984), the competent nurse has improved flexibility but may have difficulty coping with more challenging clinical issues.

The fourth stage is proficient, in which the nurse perceives situations more holistically and is guided by maxims. The fifth stage is expert, and although there is always room for improvement and continued development, the nurse has achieved a higher level of knowledge and intuition. The expert nurse has extensive experience and an intuitive grasp of complex clinical situations. (Benner, 1984). An example of an expert nurse is someone who has worked in his or her specialty for 10 to 15 years. Using this model can also be very helpful when assigning preceptors to new nurses, as mentors should be at the proficient or expert stage of knowledge development.

GROUP DYNAMICS

When you transition into your professional practice role you will be working with all types of groups. For example, every day you will work with a group of nurses and other members of the health care team. The unit you work on will have many different groups—formal and informal, large and small. The type and function of the group will certainly vary but the dynamics will be similar. Understanding the way groups work and the roles that individuals assume can be very helpful to you as you transition into your new position. Consider for a moment your past experiences working in groups. What was the purpose of the group? Was it formal or informal? Can you identify the process you engaged in when forming your group? What role did you play within the group? Were there people who monopolized the conversation? Was there a leader? Was this a positive or negative experience? Reflecting on past experiences can be quite helpful as you form new groups.

Group dynamics relate to the formation, function, structure, and process of the group (Encyclopedia.com, 2009). Groups can be formed in a formal or informal manner. For example, you may be assigned to a task force on patient education. On the other hand, you may join a group of your peers in a book club. All groups have rules or norms that relate to their structure, function, and processes. A formal task force will have a certain number of participants and meet at a specific day and time. There will be an agenda and a leader who will chair the meeting. Each member will have a specific task to complete as a member of the group. An informal group will be less structured although it will have some type of structure and processes.

The seminal work of Bruce Tuckman (1965) set the foundational framework of group formation. He described five stages of development: forming, storming, norming, performing, and adjourning. In the forming stage an orientation period occurs during which members join together and work and begin to establish the group. The next stage, the storming stage, is filled with uncertainty and conflict—there may be a positive or negative outcome. During the norming stage the members join together and become a cohesive group and the members share responsibilities and begin to see results. In the performing stage members achieve full cohesiveness and resolve their conflicts through group discussions. The final stage, adjournment, occurs when the group disbands. This may be due to conflict or because the goals of the group have been accomplished. Some groups never reach this stage as they continue to meet (Smith, 2005; Tuckman, 1965).

Your nursing unit is a group and what makes it even more complex is that the members are constantly changing. According to Tuckman's theory, there are five stages of group development: forming, storming, norming, performing, and adjourning. During these stages group members must address several issues and the way in which these issues are resolved determines whether the group will succeed in accomplishing its task (Tuckman, 1977). Each day you will work with a different group of individuals and so the group is fluid and the roles are constantly changing. Some of the roles that emerge in a group include work roles, blocking roles, and maintenance roles. Work roles include: initiator, informer, clarifier, summarizer, and reality tester. The initiator may suggest procedures. The informer shares facts and advice. The clarifier serves to interpret ideas. The summarizer restates and offers decisions. And the reality tester analyzes ideas (Encyclopedia.com, 2009). There are five maintenance roles:

- Harmonizer—reduces tensions in group
- Gatekeeper—keeps communication channels open
- Consensus tester—tests possible solutions
- Encourager—is friendly to all
- Compromiser—offers compromise

The blocking roles include:

- Aggressor—criticizes members
- Blocker—has hidden agendas and disagrees with others because of personal reasons
- Dominator—patronizes others
- Comedian—attention getters; don't do any work
- Avoidance behavior—changes topic and avoids commitment to the group (Benne & Sheats, 2007)

Groups need to establish clear roles in order to avoid role conflict and ambiguity. The overall goal is to develop a group that can overcome its differences and avoid groupthink, which occurs when a few influential members persuade people to agree with them. Group cohesiveness has many positive effects, such as job satisfaction and decreased turnover. Conversely, too much group cohesiveness can have a negative effect because the members do not want to disagree with each other. Groups also involve a certain level of trust so new members may not be accepted right away. This is true of new graduates who need to earn the trust of the other staff on the unit. It is normal to feel a bit unwelcome or at times isolated, but do not despair, with time you will be accepted into the group. Understanding the roles that individuals may play in a group can help you to become a more productive member of the group. Having a strong leader in your group is desirable as he or she has the knowledge, skills, and experience to address the negative and unproductive behavior of these group members.

LIABILITY INSURANCE

Your role as a nurse carries a certain amount of risk and you must be aware of the potential situations that may result in accusations of negligence or malpractice. The best way to avoid a legal action is to follow your Nurse Practice Act and the policies and procedures of your organization. It is also important for you to purchase your own liability or malpractice insurance because sometimes, despite our best efforts, an error will occur. Although you may also be covered under your hospital's liability plan experts agree that you should also purchase your own insurance. The cost is reasonable and if there is any type of legal action you will be protected by your policy. Many nurses believe they do not require their own insurance because they are covered under their employer's policy. However, Tammelleo (1997) posits, "An employer's policy does not provide blanket protection—there are limits to the scope, length, and amount of coverage nurses receive" (para.3). Therefore, it is highly recommended that you purchase your own policy. This way if you are involved in a lawsuit you will notify your insurance carrier who will assign legal counsel to represent your best interests. Tammelleo (1997) also recommends meeting with the risk manager at your place of employment to review the coverage you have as an employee of the organization. This will help you to figure out what type of individual policy you should purchase. There are several well-known companies that provide nurses with liability insurance. Many of these are advertised in nursing journals. You may also want to consult with your peers as to the type of policy they would recommend. One hopes you will never need to use the policy; however, it is vital to have this coverage because you never know when you might need it.

REQUIRED COURSES

All registered nurses must complete the Basic Cardiac Life Support (BCLS) course every 2 years. Most organizations provide this course for their employees either free of charge or for a nominal fee. Individual states and countries may require additional courses, so be sure to check. Some students/nurses who are interested in critical care may decide to take an advanced cardiac life support course (ACLS), or an EKG course to expand their knowledge and skills. Many courses, especially mandatory ones, will be provided by the organization. There are many certification and continuing education courses available to all nurses and whether they are mandated or not you should take as many relevant courses as possible as you are expected to be a lifelong learner. There are many continuing education courses offered online from various professional journals and organizations. Some colleges and universities also offer continuing education courses. And your own organization will most likely offer some type of professional development opportunities. Take advantage of everything as these opportunities will help you to expand your knowledge and can be added to your portfolio and résumé.

RELOCATION CULTURE IN A NEW PLACE

The job market for new-graduate nurses is highly competitive, with some areas experiencing a job shortage, whereas others experience a nurse shortage. If you live in an area that is currently experiencing a job shortage you may want to consider relocating to an area that is experiencing a nurse shortage. You may be contemplating a move to another state or to another country. Of course, moving to another country is more challenging, but certainly many new nurses do this very successfully. This decision requires careful consideration as it can be very difficult to leave loved ones and adjust to a new position and a new home. Be sure to visit the area and speak with as many people as possible. You should also make a list of pros and cons and ponder whether this will be a short-term or long-term relocation. Discuss this with your family, friends, and mentors. There are many factors you will need to consider, such as relocation costs and where you will live. You will also need to learn how to navigate your way around a new location. The culture of the area and organization you are going to work in may be very different from your own culture. There will be many adjustments and one hopes the experience will be positive. However, you will also need to have a contingency plan in case you are not happy and want to return home. It is not unusual to feel like a fish out of water when you begin a new position; hence, it is important to give yourself time to adjust to your new role. As a rule it is a good idea to stay in a position for at least a year before you make a move; this pertains to any position, whether you are working close to home or in a new location. However, if the environment is not conducive or you are very dissatisfied, then by all means you should find a new position.

SUMMARY

This chapter focused on the role of the nurse generalist and transition into professional practice. Several theoretical frameworks relating to professional development and knowledge development were also discussed. An overview of group dynamics and how they impact your role as a member of various groups was also presented. The importance of purchasing your own liability insurance was also highlighted in addition to completing any required courses for licensure.

DISCUSSION QUESTIONS

1. Describe the role of the nurse generalist.
2. Discuss the expectations of the American Colleges of Nurses and the preparation of the baccalaureate-prepared nurse.
3. Discuss the expectations of the National League for Nurses and the associate-prepared nurse.
4. Describe Kramer's stages of reality shock.
5. According to Dalton et al. (1977), what are the four stages of development employees experience?
6. List and describe Benner's (1984) stages of knowledge development.
7. How do group dynamics impact your role as a group member?
8. Why do you need to purchase your own liability insurance?
9. What course do you need to take every 2 years, at least in the United States?
10. What are some of the challenges faced when relocating for a new position?

SUGGESTED LEARNING ACTIVITIES

- Locate a copy of your state or country's Nurse Practice Act.
- Interview an advanced beginner nurse and an expert nurse and compare the differences in their experiences.
- Find three potential organizations that offer liability insurance to compare and contrast coverage and cost.

REFERENCES

American Association of Colleges of Nurses (AACN). (2008). *Essentials of baccalaureate nursing.* Retrieved from https://www.aacn.org.

American Association of Colleges of Nurses (AACN). (2014). *The impact of education on nursing practice.* Retrieved from https://www.aacn.org.

Benne, K. D., & Sheats, P. (2007). Functional Roles of Group Members. *Group Facilitation: A Research & Applications Journal, 8,* 30–35.

Benner, P. (1982). From novice to expert… the Dreyfus model of skill acquisition. *American Journal of Nursing, 82,* 402–407.

Benner, P. (1984). *From novice to expert: Excellence and power in clinical nursing practice.* Menlo CA: Addison-Wesley.

Dalton, G., Thompson, P., and Price, P. (1977). The four stages of professional careers: A new look at performance by professionals. *Organizational Dynamics, 6*(1), 23.

Dalton, G., & Thompson, P. (1986). *Novations: Strategies for career management.* Glenview, IL: Scott Foresman.

Duchscher, J. (2009). Transition shock: The initial stage of role adaptation for newly graduated Registered Nurses. *Journal of Advanced Nursing, 65*(5), 1103-1113. doi:10.1111/j.1365-2648.2008.04898.x

Encyclopedia.com. (2009). *Group dynamics.* Retrieved at https://www.encyclopedia.com

Flinter, M. (2010). *From new nurse practitioner to primary care provider: A multiple case study of new nurse practitioners who completed a formal post graduate residency training program.* (Doctoral dissertation). Storrs, CT: University of Connecticut. doi: 10.3912/OJIN.Vol17No01PPT04

Flinter, M. (2011). From new nurse practitioner to primary care provider: Bridging the transition through FQHC-based residency training. *OJIN: The Online Journal of Issues in Nursing, 17*(1). Retrieved from nursingworld.org/gm-node/39340.aspx

Kowitlawakul, Y. (2013). From novice to expert: Sharing professional development experience in different practice settings. *Singapore Nursing Journal*, *40*(3), 43–46.

Kramer, M. (1974). *Reality shock*. St. Louis, MO: Mosby.

Meleis, A. (2007). *Theoretical nursing development & progress*. New York, NY: Lippincott Williams & Wilkins.

Meleis, A., Sawyer, L., Im, E., Messias, D., & Schumacher, K. (2000). Experiencing transitions: An emerging middle-range theory. *Advances in Nursing Science*, *23*(1), 12–28.

National League for Nursing. (2013). *Competencies of the associate degree nurse*. Retrieved from https://www.nln.org

New York State Education Department Office of the Professions. (2010). *Education law, article 139, nursing*. Retrieved from https://www.op.nysed.gov/prof/nurse/article139.htm

Professional liability insurance program for nurse professionals. (2007). *Wyoming Nurse*, *20*(3), 6–8

Smith, M. K. (2005). *Bruce W. Tuckman—Forming, storming, norming and performing in groups, the encyclopaedia of informal education*. Retrieved from http://infed.org/mobi/bruce-w-tuckman-forming-storming-norming-and-performing-in-groups

Tammelleo, A. (1997). Legally speaking. Malpractice insurance: For your protection. *RN*, *60*(10), 73.

Tuckman, B. W. (1965). Developmental sequence in small groups. *Psychological Bulletin*, *63*, 384–399.

Tuckman, B. W., & Jensen, M. C. (1977). Stages of small-group development revisited. *Group & Organization Studies*, *2*(4), 419–427.

Tyrell-Smith, T. (2011 February 15). Four stages of a successful career. *US News and World Report*. Retrieved from https://www.money.usnews.com/.../15/four-stages-of-a-successful-career

CHAPTER 10

Strategies for Successful Transition

Success is not final, failure is not fatal: it is the courage to continue that counts.

—Winston Churchill

OBJECTIVES

At the end of this chapter the reader will be able to:

- Describe the transition strategies for new graduates
- Describe the orientation process for new graduates
- Identify time-management and organization strategies
- Describe the role of preceptors, mentors, nurse managers, and staff development
- Describe nurse manager staff development
- Understand the relationship of job satisfaction and turnover
- Discuss the key aspects of the National Council of State Boards of Nursing (NCSBN) tips for transition

The day has finally arrived and you are ready to begin the next phase of your incredible journey into the world of professional nursing. This day will come for all of you and when it does you will be filled with excitement, anticipation, and some trepidation because of the uncertainty inherent in this new experience. The transition process is challenging for most and smooth sailing for some. Due to the myriad issues involved in this transition, most of you will begin your new career with a formal orientation period. The length of this orientation will vary; however, the goal of the orientation program is similar as it is meant to help you acclimate into your new work environment. During your formal orientation you will learn all about the organization and about your specific role within the organization. You will spend some time in the classroom, however, most of the time in the clinical area will be spent with a preceptor to guide you through the process. You will meet many people along the way; some will help you and some will hinder you, but you will learn something from each and every one of them. Beginning a new job, especially as a new nurse, can be very overwhelming; however, there are strategies, such as time management and organizational skills, that you develop to address some of the challenges you will face. This chapter will provide you with valuable strategies for your transition.

TRANSITION STRATEGIES

The transition process of new-graduate nurses is one fraught with challenges, trials and tribulations, and mastery of content. The new graduate typically begins the transition process eager with anticipation and hope. Unfortunately, many new graduates find the transition process to be challenging at best and totally overwhelming at worst. According to Baxter (2010), many new graduates are so dissatisfied with their experience that they leave the job within the first year, resulting in attrition rate of 60%. There are numerous factors that affect the transition and it is difficult to isolate them. These factors include lack of educational preparation (Duchscher, 2008), self-doubt, anxiety, reality shock, preceptor issues, and inadequate orientation. "NGNs (new-graduate nurses) often face unwelcoming clinical environments, high patient acuity, and advanced medical technology" (Baxter, 2010, p. E12). You may not have control over all the factors; however, you can learn how to advocate for yourself and take control of your own destiny. Duchscher (2008) described a process of transition in which new graduates advance through the stages of doing—learning the role and completing assignments—understanding the rationale, and knowing—the "a-ha!" moment. She based this theory of transition on new-graduate nurses who were not let licensed. Interestingly, Gerrish (2000) found that new graduates were better equipped to transition than they had been in the past. This may be due to the fact that most organizations have improved and lengthened their formal orientation programs. Some health care organizations hire new-graduate nurses prior to completion of their licensure exam. In this type of situation the new graduate must work with her or his preceptor until the licensure exam is passed, thus this process may not be applicable to all new-graduate nurses. Nonetheless, new graduates all experience a transition process. You may not have control over all the factors, however, you can learn how to advocate for yourself and take control of your own destiny. There are several strategies that address some of the challenges that new graduates may face during their transition. Rush et al. (2013) concluded that new graduates require more education on practical skills, 6 to 9 months of support, socialization with peers, healthy work environments, and preceptors who have been formally prepared.

There is a dearth of literature on the benefits of positive thinking, thus developing a mindset in which you envision your success can be very helpful. Positive thinking is also related to hopeful thinking. Schudson (1999) posits that people are hopeful about multiple things, such as new positions and new beginnings. He further states that hope does not just happen, but that people work hard to keep hope alive. Positive thinking is related to being happy and successful and can have a great impact on your life (Collins, 2009). Positive thinking is also related to patient healing (Power of Positive Thinking, 2002). Beginning your new position with positive intentions for success can be very powerful. People who demonstrate a positive attitude may influence others to adopt a similar attitude. Try to envision yourself in the role as you hope to experience it, however, try to be realistic in your thinking. If you set your goals too high you may be disappointed if you cannot achieve them. You may want to set an overall goal and then set a daily intention and goal for the day. Try to focus on the present and break things down into smaller steps; with each small success your confidence will increase.

SELF-CARE

Transitioning to your professional practice role is quite stressful. Self-care is a very effective way to decrease stress and should be used throughout one's personal and professional journey. There are many strategies that can be used (see Chapter 3) and you should try to integrate these into your daily rituals. Deep breathing and relaxation techniques are easy to do and are very useful in the clinical area. You might want to start your day with a moment of silence and six deep cleansing breaths. Then throughout the day whenever you are feeling stress or anxiety you can repeat the exercise. This will help you to become grounded and you will then be able to focus on the task at hand. It is also important to get enough sleep because when you are tired you are more likely to be stressed. You will need your energy to sustain you throughout a 12-hour shift. Working a 12-hour shift is exhausting and this may be a big adjustment because many clinical rotations are only 6 or 8 hours in length. Following a healthy nutrition plan and engaging in physical activity are also very important. If you are working on the day shift be sure to eat a healthy breakfast and lunch. Conversely, if you are on the night shift you will want to eat a healthy dinner. Adjusting to the night shift is also a challenge and as a new graduate there is a good chance you will be working 12-hour night shifts. If you do work the night shift you will have to figure out a sleeping schedule. It will take time but eventually your body will adjust and you will develop a healthy sleeping pattern. Resting and sleeping are vital for your health and well-being, thus you will want to employ strategies such as meditation and decreasing caffeine intake, and perhaps drinking some chamomile tea before bedtime. You will also spend hours standing and walking so it is vital to have comfortable shoes and to elevate your legs throughout the day. Embracing a healthy lifestyle with proper nutrition, rest, and physical activity will serve you well, and you will be a positive role model for your patients.

SELF-ADVOCACY

Most of us have a difficult time self-advocating, and the task is even more challenging for a new nurse; however, you must learn how to become your own advocate. You will need to become more assertive. Assertiveness means being able to communicate with others in a way that enables one to express his or her rights without demeaning others (Ünal, 2012). Ünal (2012) described a study on student nurses who completed a course in assertiveness training and found that self-esteem improved as assertiveness increased. If you have a conflict with your preceptor or one of the staff on your unit you will need to address the conflict. If you do not address the situation it will most likely get worse. You need to let your preceptor and staff development instructor know about your learning needs. Perhaps you feel you need more education regarding the electronic medical records, or how to perform a certain procedure. Or you might feel that they are advancing you too quickly. Whatever the issue you will need to share this with your preceptor, staff development instructor, and nurse manager. Admittedly this can be difficult; however, it is to your benefit. It is a good idea to write down your thoughts on paper and if you are really nervous you may want to role play with someone prior to your actual conversation. You want to be assertive but not abrasive so choose your words wisely. There will be many times when you will need to self-advocate and after you get over your initial fear you will feel empowered to continue to do so.

GOALS

It can be very helpful to develop daily or weekly goals as you transition into your professional practice role. Achieving goals can be very motivating and also helps to build your confidence. As a new nurse you may want to develop an overall goal for the week with a small daily goal that relates to your overall goal. For example, you may develop a goal relating to stress management. Your weekly goal could be to meditate for 5 minutes per day by the end of the week. Each day you would set a small goal you intend to achieve, for example, practice deep breathing and relaxation for at least 1 minute on days one and two, and then on days three and four your goal would be to meditate for 2 minutes. On days five and six you would increase your meditation to 4 minutes and then on day seven you would try for the entire 5 minutes. Another weekly goal could be to be able to perform a certain task independently, or to work on time management. There are myriad goals you can develop for yourself. You can write them in your journal or on your computer. A template (Table 10.1) has been provided for you to use when developing your goals. It is also important to reward yourself when you reach your goals. This might be a positive accolade or treating yourself to something special—a small present, a 10-minute massage, or lunch with friends. You can decide at the beginning of the week how you will reward yourself when you reach your goals. Just be careful not to get upset if you don't reach your goal. If you reach it great, if not, try again the following week. Perhaps you set the bar too high, so try to be a bit more realistic and set an achievable goal. It is great to challenge yourself but you don't want to set yourself up for failure by being too ambitious.

TABLE 10.1
Template for Weekly Transition Goals

Weekly Goals	
Week: _____	Goal for the Week: _____
Daily Goals (activities performed to achieve weekly goal)	
Monday: _____	Completed: _____
Tuesday: _____	Completed: _____
Wednesday: _____	Completed: _____
Thursday: _____	Completed: _____
Friday: _____	Completed: _____
Saturday: _____	Completed: _____
Sunday: _____	Completed: _____
Reward: _____	
Lessons Learned: _____	

SUPPORT GROUPS

Support groups are very helpful for new nurses and if there is one available in your organization you should try to attend. You might also make a suggestion to your organization to develop a support group. These groups can be very helpful and provide a safe environment for you to discuss challenges, accomplishments or frustrations. Venting can be very therapeutic and just talking about an issue can be very helpful. Members can share strategies and techniques for handling difficult situations. Members can also celebrate milestones and achievements. Even if there is no formal support group you might participate in an informal group with some of your peers and coworkers. Oftentimes, the nurses and other new employees you meet during the hospital-wide orientation will become your support group as you all share a special bond as new members of the organization. This type of support can also be very helpful, although it will lack the guidance of a nonbiased moderator. Your friends and family will be there to support you through your transition, so do not despair if you do not have access to a support group.

ORIENTATION PROCESS

The orientation process is part and parcel of your successful transition. Health care organizations that are accredited by The Joint Commission must adhere to standards regarding hiring and training of personnel. You may visit the website for additional information. Today many organizations realize the significance of a well-developed orientation. According to Robitaille (2013), "an effective orientation process is crucial to help ensure an individual's competency to perform his or her role and to familiarize the orientee with an organization's culture, policies and procedures, and unit-level protocols" (p. C7). Orientation consists of didactic and clinical experiences with the average length of time for a new graduate being 3 to 6 months. According to Duchscher (2008), "Graduates require consistency, predictability, stability, and familiarity in their initial clinical practice situations for at least the first 4 months" (p. 448). Baxter (2010) described the lack of research regarding the ideal length of time for orientation with programs varying from 12 weeks to 18 months in length and the average being 12 weeks. Intuitively, one would think that the longer the orientation the better, which may be true but the quality of the program is just as important.

All orientation programs vary with the orientee being expected to achieve core competencies by the end of the orientation period. Orientation usually begins with the didactic part, which includes classes about the organization; mandatory courses, such as fire safety and infection control; and related policies and procedures. Technology training will also be included if the organization uses an electronic medical record. Many organizations also include simulation experiences. During this phase of orientation you will come in contact with the various administrators. As mentioned, you will also form a bond with the other new employees. Many organizations hold general orientations during which all disciplines attend classes and then have break-out sessions to cover specific material based on discipline. In general the nursing orientation tends to be more comprehensive as your role is highly complex.

The clinical piece is done on a more individualized basis and most often a preceptor is assigned to mentor you throughout the duration of your clinical orientation. Depending on your specialty you may continue to attend some didactic classes throughout your orientation. For example, you may need to complete a critical care course, respiratory course, or another type of course related to your specialty. Many organizations require you to begin your nursing career on a medical/surgical unit; however, there are some hospitals, especially ones that offer residency programs that may hire new graduates into various specialty areas. Naturally, these require an extensive orientation program. Nursing leaders and educators have conflicting opinions regarding new nurses working in a specialty area. Some believe all new graduates should begin their nursing careers on medical–surgical units, whereas others disagree. There is no need to limit yourself, the real key is to find a position in which you will be provided with the education and support required of all new-graduate nurses regardless of the unit to which they are assigned. However, the vacancy rates in medical/surgical units are usually higher than in other areas. According to a recent report by Nursing Solutions (2014), the highest rate of turnover was in med–surg with a national turnover rate of 24% followed by the emergency department with a rate of 20.3%. The lowest rate of turnover was 10% in surgical services.

Many nurses begin their careers in medical/surgical units and then transition to a specialty area. This is a wonderful way to gain experience and to acquire the foundational knowledge required for working in a specialty unit.

The orientation is a formalized process and you will most likely be provided with a comprehensive schedule. There will be expectations, goals and objectives, and required competencies. The clinical orientation is progressive in nature and you will continue to become more autonomous as the weeks go by. You will work with your preceptor and share the clinical assignment. The pattern usually begins with an observation and then you advance from a modified assignment all the way up to a complete patient assignment. Throughout this time you will be evaluated on your performance. The key people in this process are the preceptor, staff development instructor, nurse manager, and mentor. Some programs are more formal, with weekly team meetings, whereas others only meet formally a few times throughout the program. You may also request a meeting if you desire one. When you begin your orientation program you will be provided with a list of contacts and their roles within the organization. Organizations understand the importance of organizational support for new employees (Baxter, 2010). To that end they invest time and money into your orientation and truly want you to be successful, so be sure to use all the resources that are available.

Some organizations follow a specific framework for their orientation programs. The competency-based orientation (CBO) was developed by Fey and Miltner (2000). This framework requires the orientee to achieve a list of competencies throughout the orientation period (Baxter, 2010). Some programs use Benner's (1980) novice-to-expert framework to guide the development of their programs, which are based on adult learning theories and include reflective practice (Baxter, 2010). Another framework is based on critical pathways and is used to guide orientation in a specialty area (Baxter, 2010). The framework is certainly important, however, active participation and consistency are key. You need to take an active role in your orientation so that you can demonstrate your potential and competency development. Following the program, being assigned one consistent preceptor (an alternate may be needed to cover unplanned days off) and orientating on your assigned shift and unit are also important.

PRECEPTORS AND MENTORS

Preceptors

Preceptors play a vital role in the orientation of new-graduate nurses (Baxter, 2010; Hoffart et al., 2011). A preceptor and a mentor are different and you need to have both of these supports.

A preceptor is a specially trained nurse who is paired up with you and helps guide your clinical orientation experience. Ideally, the preceptor should complete formal training and be given a lighter assignment so he or she can spend adequate time with you (Baxter, 2010). Most often you will have one main preceptor for the duration of your clinical orientation. However, if you are being assigned to the night shift you will complete the first part of your orientation on the day shift and the rest of it on the night shift. Naturally, you will be assigned a different preceptor on the night shift. Preceptors should volunteer for the role or they may not be very supportive. Ideally, preceptors will have 2 to 4 years of clinical experience as they are better able to simplify things than an expert nurse (Benner, 1980, as cited in Baxter, 2010). The preceptor plays a vital role in your successful transition so it is important to develop a strong relationship with this person. Unfortunately, some new nurses do have issues with their preceptors and it is important for you to take a proactive approach if you are having such difficulties. Strategies for addressing issues relating to your preceptor will be discussed in Chapter 14. With luck, you will be assigned a preceptor who will be knowledgeable and supportive and know how to balance your assignment.

Mentors

Mentors are different from preceptors; however, they do provide invaluable support throughout your career. All students and nurses should have a mentor. Although there are some programs that match new nurses with mentors most nurses locate their own mentors.

Finding a mentor can be challenging and before you make a formal request of someone you should figure out what you hope to gain from this relationship. Some examples of mentors are faculty members, nurse managers, senior staff nurses, and—once you are finished with your orientation—your preceptor may become your mentor. Some organizations have developed formal mentoring programs. For example, some nursing schools have peer mentoring programs, which are beneficial while you are navigating your way through your academic program. Mills and Mullins (2008) described a formal mentoring program that was piloted in California. The purpose of this program was to offer guidance, assistance, and support to new nurses with the expected outcomes being quality of care, nurse job satisfaction, and decreased turnover. The pilot program was very successful with both the mentors and the new nurses being very satisfied.

A mentor is someone who actively advises, guides, and promotes another's career and training. The mentor and protégé develop a strong connection and the mentor may guide the protégé in professional, academic, and personal decisions (Vance, 1982, 2010). Many individuals have different mentors for various purposes at different times of their lives. "Mentors provide informal support by answering questions and giving encouragement and feedback" (Baxter, 2010, p. E14).

Williams and Grant (2012) described the attributes of a mentor, which include the ability to manage the mentor–protégé relationship, and nurture, respect, teach, encourage, and support the mentee/protégé. Furthermore, mentors should be empathetic, nonjudgmental, honest, and have good listening skills. Mentors are especially helpful to the new graduate in transition. "Good mentorship relationships aid thinking, reasoning, problem-solving and encourage questions about aspects of patient care. This prepares nursing students for the kind of experiential learning and development that is needed throughout their careers" (Hodges, 2009, p. 32). The mentor should have time available to meet with his or her protégé and to keep appointments and vice versa.

The attributes described above are the types of qualities you will want to seek in your mentors. You will also want to avoid selecting the wrong type of mentor, such as the "toxic mentor" (Vance, 2010; Clutterbuck, 2004), who is more concerned with his or her own issues and may be aggressive and have a hidden agenda. Because this is a relationship you will also need certain behaviors so that you can have a positive relationship with your mentor. For example, you need to be committed to the relationship and be honest and open to the sage advice of your mentor. This is not to say that you need to follow all the suggestions of your mentor, but you should consider them. You also need to be respectful of your mentor and the time and effort he or she is putting into this relationship.

There are all types of mentoring relationships, with some requiring a formal contract and others just a verbal agreement. Developing a contract or formal agreement can be beneficial as both parties will know exactly what is expected of them.

A mentor is someone you should be able to consult with when you need advice. The mentor cannot make decisions for you, but he or she can help you to make an informed decision. Glynn and Silva (2013) described the benefits of a nurse internship for new nurses in critical care. The internship provides a combination of didactic and clinical experiences with support from the preceptor and a clinical nurse specialist. New nurses can make a successful transition into a specialty area as long as they complete an internship/residency or fellowship program. Typically, these types of programs last 1 year and are highly competitive. You will also be expected to read and study and take exams throughout the year. Some parts will be similar to nursing school, so you must be prepared for this type of intensive experience, however, it will be well worth your effort.

The mentor relationship often goes through a process of stages with the first stage being getting acquainted with your mentor and developing your relationship and ground rules. The next stage is the working stage during which the mentor is formally supporting and guiding you. The final stage is the closure stage, which may end formally, informally, or continue for many years (Williams & Grant, 2012).

TIME MANAGEMENT AND ORGANIZATIONAL SKILLS

Two of the biggest challenges you will face throughout your transition will be to develop time management and organizational skills. Even if you believe you are an organized person, working on a busy unit requires a high level of organization and time management. Developing these skills evolves over time, however, there are strategies that you may employ to improve both of these vital skills. Mitchell et al. (2010) identify these as soft skills, which may not be focused on during your student days, but are extremely important and may be a critical factor in the hiring process in addition to enabling a smooth transition. Certainly, your preceptor and mentor can serve as role models and help you to develop your time management and organizational skills. White (2013) recommends the following strategies for improving time management:

- Make a list
- Set deadlines
- Stop multitasking
- Delegate responsibilities
- Use your downtime
- Reward yourself

These strategies will also help you become more organized. Strategies for helping to foster organizational skills include developing goals, making lists, and prioritizing your tasks. Time management and organizational skills develop as you are progressing through your orientation. Caring for a complex patient assignment will require good organizational skills. For example, having the appropriate tools to do your job is vital. Every day you need to bring your stethoscope, pens, penlight, small notebook, or personal digital assistant (PDA) (if it is allowed), so you can start your day right. When you are ready to assess your patients at the beginning of the shift think about what you need to complete this task. This way you will not waste time running back and forth for equipment. You should have learned this as a student; however, you will need to develop your organizational skills. Whenever you are preparing to care for your patients think about what you have to do and what equipment you may need to complete the task. Of course, there are many factors that may cause you to be delayed as the status of your patients can be unpredictable. Sometimes even the most organized nurses have a day that is chaotic and disorganized. However, with good time management and organizational skills you should be able to accomplish everything you need to during your shift. Another way to improve your skills is to complete a self-assessment of your soft skills. This way you can identify areas for improvement and develop specific goals.

JOB SATISFACTION

Job satisfaction is a very important predictor of turnover and/or job retention. Lynn, Morgan, and Moore (2009) define job satisfaction as "the extent to which a nurse is satisfied with his or her workload and the colleagues with whom he or she works" (p. 9).There are many factors that influence a nurse's job satisfaction such as autonomy, supervisor support, and work environment (Aiken et al., 2001; Bratt et al., 2000; Davidson, Folcarelli, Crawford, Duprat, & Clifford, 1997; Lee et al., 1996). New nurses often have high rates of turnover with reports as high as 50% to 70% (Kovner et al., 2007). They are not satisfied with their roles due to the overwhelming challenges they face during the transition. However, when new nurses are in a supportive environment and complete a preceptor-based orientation their job satisfaction increases and retention rates increase (Almada et al., 2008). In support of this Beecroft, Dorey, and Wenton (2008) found that turnover rates decreased when new nurses had increased job satisfaction. Therefore, it is important to seek employment in organizations that have well-developed orientation programs and ongoing support. Unfortunately, you may not have this option but it is certainly important to keep in mind as you are searching for your first position.

NCSBN'S TRANSITION TO PRACTICE MODEL

It is a well-known fact that new nurses face many challenges as they transition into professional practice. In an effort to address this crucial situation The National Council of State Boards of Nursing (NCSBN, 2014) developed the Transition to Practice model (TTP) citing the need for best practices for training new nurses and for decreasing turnover rates. Some of the issues highlighted by the NCSBN (2014) that guided the development of this model include three main problem and impact issues. The first problem is that new nurses care for sicker patients in complex health systems, with the impact being that 40% of new nurses have made a medication error. The next problem is that new nurses have high levels of stress, which is related to patient safety and practice errors. The third problem is that approximately 25% of new nurses leave their profession within the first year. The TTP is currently being piloted in Illinois, North Carolina, and Ohio and is currently in Phase 2. The results of this pilot will be discussed at the NCSBN's annual meeting in August 2014. Based on the results a decision will be made on the merits of this model and on whether or not to implement it across the country.

The TTP consists of the following modules:

- Preceptor Training
- Patient Centered Care
- Communication and Teamwork
- Evidence-based Practice
- Quality Improvement
- Informatics

These modules, with the exception of preceptor training, are the same topics that are included in Quality and Safety Education for Nurses (QSEN) competencies. Developing a model for a standardized transition of new nurses is an excellent idea and it is to be hoped that it will have a positive impact on new-nurse transition and quality of care.

Top 10 Tips for Your First Year of Transition

1. Think positively.
2. Develop weekly goals.
3. Find a mentor.
4. Engage in self-care.
5. Advocate for yourself.
6. Improve your time-management and organizational skills.
7. Apply for internships/residencies/fellowships.
8. Try to select an organization with a comprehensive orientation program.
9. Be an active participant in your orientation.

SUMMARY

This chapter focused on strategies for a successful transition. An overview of transition strategies was provided. The orientation process was described; included in this discussion was the role of preceptors and mentors. The importance of soft skills, such as time management and organization, was also included. Job satisfaction and its relationship to turnover were briefly discussed and an overview of the NCSBN's TTP model, being piloted in three states, was described.

DISCUSSION QUESTIONS

1. List and describe three transition strategies.
2. What is the role of the preceptor?
3. Describe the role of the mentor.
4. What are the different types of orientation programs?
5. List three ways you can improve time management.
6. List three ways you can improve organizational skills.
7. What are some factors that are related to job satisfaction?
8. What is the Transition to Practice model?
9. What are some self-care strategies you can employ?
10. Why is self-advocacy important?

SUGGESTED LEARNING ACTIVITIES

- Explore opportunities/requirements for internships and fellowships.
- Complete a self-assessment of your soft skills.
- Consider what you would like in a mentor and list at least three individuals who could serve as your mentor. After you develop a guide for what you would like your mentor to help you with invite one of your three choices to be your mentor.
- Write an essay about the NCSBN's Transition to Practice model.

REFERENCES

Aiken, L., Clarke, S., Sloane, D., Pachulski, J., Busse, R., Clark, H.,...Shamian, J. (2001). Nurses reports on hospital care in five countries. *Health Affairs, 2*(3), 43–60.

Almada, P., Carafoli, K., Flattery, J.B., French, D.A., & McNamara, M. (2004). Improving the retention of newly graduated nurses. *Journal for Nurses in Staff Development, 20*(6), 268–273.

Baxter, P. (2010). Providing orientation programs to new graduate nurses: Points to consider. *Journal for Nurses in Staff Development, 26*(4), E12–E17. doi:10.1097/NND.0b013e3181d80319

Beecroft, P., Dorey. F., & Wenten, M., (2008). Turnover intention in new graduate nurses: a multivariate analysis. *Journal of Advanced Nursing, 62*(1), 41–52.

Bratt, M., Broome, M., Kelber, S., & Lostocco, L. (2000). Influence of stress and nursing leadership on job satisfaction of pediatric intensive care unit nurses. *American Journal of Critical Care, 9*(5), 307–317.

Clutterbuck, D. (2004). Everyone needs a mentor. *CIPD.*

Collins, G. (2010). *The impact of positive thinking.* Retrieved from http://EzineArticles.com/?expert=Greg_J_Collins

Davidson, H., Folcarelli, P., Crawford, S., Duprat, L., & Clifford, J. (1997). The effects of health care reforms on job satisfaction and voluntary turnover among hospital based nurses. *Medical Care, 35*(6), 634–645.

Duchscher, J. (2008). A process of becoming: The stages of new nursing graduate professional role transition. *Journal of Continuing Education in Nursing, 39*(10), 441–450. doi: 10.3928/00220124- 20081001-03.

Fey, M. K., & Miltner, R. S. (2000). A competency-based orientation program for new graduate nurses. *Journal of Nursing Administration, 30*(3), 126–132.

Gerrish, K. (2000). Still fumbling along? A comparative study of the newly qualified nurse's perception of the transition from student to qualified nurse. *Journal of Advanced Nursing, 32*(2), 473–480. doi:10.1046/j.1365-2648.2000.01498.x

Glynn, P., & Silva, S. (2013). Meeting the needs of new graduates in the emergency department: A qualitative study evaluating a new graduate internship program. *JEN: Journal of Emergency Nursing, 39*(2), 173–178. doi:10.1016/j.jen.2011.10.007

Hodges, B. (2009). Factors that can influence mentorship relationships. *Paediatric Nursing, 21*(6), 32–35.

Hoffart, N., Waddell, A., & Young, M. B. (2011). A model of new nurse transition. *Journal of Professional Nursing, 27*(6), 334–343. doi:10.1016/j.profnurs.2011.04.011

Kovner, C., Brewer, C., Fairchild, S., Poornima, S., Kim, H., & Djukic, M. (2007). Newly licensed RNs' characteristics, work attitudes, and intentions to work. *American Journal of Nursing, 107*(9), 58–70.

Lee, T., Mitchell, T., Wise, L., & Fireman, S. (1996). An unfolding model of voluntary employee turnover. *Academy of Management Journal, 39*(1), 5–36.

Leong, J., & Crossman, J. (2009). What nursing managers need to know: Role-transition for newly qualified nurses in Singapore. *Singapore Nursing Journal, 36*(2), 28–34.

Lynn, M., Morgan, J., & Moore, K. (2009). Development and testing of the satisfaction in nursing scale. *Nursing Research, 58*(3), 166–174.

Mills, J., & Mullins, A. (2008). The California Nurse Mentor Project: Every nurse deserves a mentor. *Nursing Economic$, 26*(5), 310–315.

Mitchell, G.W., Skinner, L.B., & White, B.J. (2010). Essential soft skills for success in the twenty-first century workforce as perceived by business educators. *Delta Pi Epsilon Journal, 52*(1), 43–53.

Nursing Solutions. (2014). *2014 National Healthcare & RN Retention Report.* Retrieved from www.nsinursingsolutions.com/.../NationalHealthcare-RNRetentionReport2

Power of positive thinking. (2002). *IIE Solutions, 34*(6), 66.

Robitaille, P. (2013). Preceptor-based orientation programs for new nurse graduates. *AORN Journal, 98*(5), C7–8. doi:10.1016/S0001-2092(13)01080-6.

Rush, K. L., Adamack, M., Gordon, J., Lilly, M., & Janke, R. (2013). Best practices of formal new graduate nurse transition programs: An integrative review. *International Journal of Nursing Studies, 50*(3), 345–356. doi:10.1016/j.ijnurstu.2012.06.009

Schudson, M. (1999). You've got mail: A few observations on hope. *Social Research, 66*(2), 625–628.

Ünal, S. (2012). Evaluating the effect of self-awareness and communication techniques on nurses' assertiveness and self-esteem. *Contemporary Nurse: A Journal for the Australian Nursing Profession, 43*(1), 90–98. doi:10.5172/conu.2012.43.1.90

Vance, C. (1982). The mentor connection. *Journal of Nursing Administration, 12*(4), 7–13.

Vance, C. (2010). *Fast facts for career success in nursing: Making the most of mentoring in a nutshell.* New York, NY: Springer Publishing.

White, D. (2013). 6 Tips to Improve Your Time Management Skills. *Psych Central.* Retrieved on March 18, 2014, from http://psychcentral.com/lib/6-tips-to-improve-your-time-management-skills/00015735

Williams, Z., & Grant, A. (2012). How to be a good mentor. *Education for Primary Care, 23*(1), 56–58.

CHAPTER 11

Clinical Practice

The most important practical lesson that can be given to nurses is to teach them what to observe.

—Florence Nightingale

OBJECTIVES

At the end of this chapter, the reader will be able to:

- Identify key aspects of the nurse generalist's role
- Understand the significance of clinical competency
- Describe professionalism in relation to role
- Understand the significance of teamwork and collaboration
- Describe cultural issues in the health care setting
- Understand his or her role as a patient advocate
- Describe patient safety and quality of care

During the first 2 years of your transition into professional practice you will be applying the theoretical and clinical concepts you learned as a nursing student. As previously discussed you will begin this role as an advanced beginner (Benner, 1984), although you may still be a novice (Benner, 1984) in areas where you did not have adequate preparation. When you graduate from your nursing program you have the foundations on which to build. Therefore, during the next 2 years you will continue to develop your role as a nurse generalist. You will also need to demonstrate proficiency and competence in a wide array of clinical competencies. The orientation and transition are geared toward helping you to achieve these requirements. There are many aspects of your role that may have only been briefly reviewed in your nursing program. Furthermore, every organization is unique so you may need to relearn some of the policies and procedures you have previously been taught. This chapter will provide more details in some of the important areas that inform and impact your role as a registered professional nurse.

ROLES AND RESPONSIBILITIES IN CLINICAL PRACTICE

The roles and responsibilities in clinical practice will be somewhat variable based on the type of health care organization and unit on which you will be working. Clinical practice can take place within a hospital, community, or health care agency in patients across the life span with a plethora of illnesses. Although these settings are different and will require various types of nursing care they also have similarities. For example, you will be using the nursing process in all of these settings. You will also be focused on health and wellness promotion and teaching your patients how to manage their health. Every day you will strive to deliver quality care and promote positive patient outcomes. You will also be serving as a patient advocate and collaborating with the interprofessional team. Theisen and Sandau (2013) identified psychomotor critical thinking as the two most important areas that nursing students must rapidly master. There are so many areas you will be developing; however, many of these were experienced as a novice—you are now in the advanced beginner role (Benner, 1980).

The nursing process is widely embraced in nursing and was originally developed by Orlando in 1958. The steps include assessment, planning, interventions, and evaluation and the process is used extensively. "It is a conceptual framework that allows a systematic evaluation of a patient's current health status and needs" (Huckabay, 2009, as cited in Lubbe & Roets, 2014, p. 60). Assessment falls under the scope of practice for registered professional nurses. However, in a recent study that was conducted in South Africa, Lubbe and Roets (2014) found that 80% of risk assessments were performed by nurses who were not licensed to do assessments. This is a serious issue as it is related to poor quality of care. The findings of the assessment influence the plan of care so it is vital to have a competent nurse complete the assessment. For example, Lubbe and Roets (2014) described pressure ulcers risk assessment and how it is an important competency for all nurses and new graduates to use the scale correctly. Assessing your patients, whether they are inpatient, outpatient, in a critical care or medical–surgical unit, is one of the most important things you will do as a nurse and you will continue to develop your assessment skills every day. According to Austin (2008) "the five steps of the nursing process are recognized as a universal approach to nursing practice" (p. 35), and include assessment, nursing diagnosis, planning, implementation, and evaluation. A template for a brief head-to-toe assessment (known as the 5-minute assessment) is included in the Appendix. As a new nurse you will have to hone your skills and with time and repetition you will become more competent. Certainly your preceptor will be helping you with this and other clinical skills. Planning and interventions will also be a priority and evaluating and revising your plan must be done on a continual basis.

Learning how to prioritize care requires critical thinking and reasoning (Theisen & Sandau, 2013). One of the biggest challenges new nurses face is to manage a group of patients as this is very different from caring for two patients under the supervision and guidance of a clinical instructor or preceptor. When you have a group of four to six patients or more you need to prioritize who needs to be taken care of first. If all of them are stable, then you can proceed in a systematic manner. Oftentimes your patients will be in a district or in consecutive rooms so you can start in one room and continue from room to room until you are finished. However, there are times when one or two are unstable so you need to prioritize. You will need to use your critical-thinking skills, problem-solving skills, and your existing knowledge about the disease process and the unique needs of your patients. Certainly, you will use the ABCs (airway, breathing, and circulation). For example, if you are assigned six patients and one is experiencing dyspnea you must assess and treat that patient first. As a new nurse it is easy to be so hyper focused on completing your initial assessments that you may not consider which patient needs your immediate attention. However, this is a vital skill and you must continue to learn how to prioritize your time.

Maslow's hierarchy of needs (see Figure 11.1) can be very helpful in guiding your assessment and prioritization in regard to prioritizing your patients as a whole and considering the individual needs of the patient. According to McCleod (2007), Maslow (1943, 1954) developed the original model to understand what motivates people. Although this is a behavioral theory it certainly has applications in the clinical arena and may be used as a guide when meeting the needs of patients/families. Looking at the model you will see that the most important needs are on the bottom of the triangle. Physiological needs

FIGURE 11.1 Maslow's Hierarchy of Needs

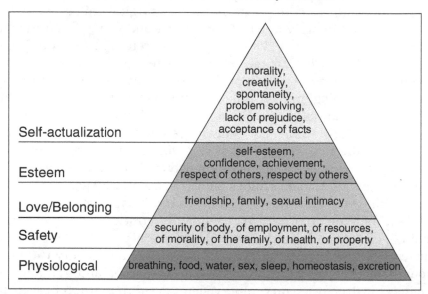

include breathing, food, water, sleep, sex, homeostasis, and excretion. Next on the triangle are safety needs such as protection and security. As nurses we are always focused on the safety of our patients. This is why it is important to develop a system for assessment, such as the one that is included at the end of this chapter. Love/Belonging is next on the list and although it is important for patients to have their family members present the bigger priority is to meet their physiological needs first. Self-esteem is next and you can meet the needs of your patients by being respectful and delivering patient-centered care. Self-actualization relates to developing self-fulfillment, which is unique to each individual; this level may never be achieved. Providing holistic patient-centered can help you to meet the patient's needs and prioritize care.

Learning how to prioritize can be challenging, nonetheless it is an integral part of your nursing role. Remember this will take time so be sure to consult with your preceptor, instructor, manager, mentor, and experienced nurses on your unit.

The acuity and number of patients you are assigned will greatly impact your ability to prioritize and complete your assignment. The nurse/patient ratio, which has been extensively addressed in the literature, varies based on the organization, geographic location, and type of unit. Evidence does support the relationship between staffing ratios and patient mortality. However, what is lacking is the evidence related to best practices in actual ratios. For example, a 6:1 ratio in medical–surgical units is common, however, some organizations have implemented a 5:1 or 4:1 ratio. Intuitively one could reason that a smaller nurse:patient ratio would lead to improved patient outcomes and decreased mortality, however, research is needed to identify best practices (Shekelle, 2013). Some states and countries have mandated staffing guidelines, or agreements with their bargaining unit, although this issue is fraught with controversy over whether it is best to have staffing guidelines or mandated staffing ratios. Some experts believe that one must consider acuity and other factors and staffing ratios may be too rigid (Allen, 2013), although in the states that have instituted mandatory staffing ratios, such as California, the results have been favorable and include decreased burnout, reduced workload, and fewer deaths (Allen, 2013). Ideally, you should have explored this when selecting your place of employment.

CLINICAL COMPETENCY AND PERFORMANCE EVALUATIONS

The Joint Commission (TJC) has standards relating to competency and the American Nurses Association (ANA) also supports competency as a professional standard (Theisen & Sandau, 2013). Nurses must demonstrate clinical competence when they begin their nursing roles in an organization whether they are a new graduate or experienced nurse, albeit an experienced nurse will be able to demonstrate these competencies in a more timely fashion. Clinical competency is a broad term used to define expectations related to clinical skills, critical thinking, problem solving, and understanding and implementation of a wide array of policies and procedures. Clinical competency statements may include performance expectations in the psychomotor, affective, and cognitive domains. Some organizations have their nurses complete a self-assessment and use that as a guide to individualize the orientation. As the nurse progresses through the orientation he or she is observed performing various tasks and will be deemed competent or not. If not, they will be given further instruction and practice and observed again. The expectation is that nurses will achieve the competencies by the end of the orientation period. As per The Joint Commission (2014) nurses must demonstrate competency and be evaluated annually. A competency checklist with performance expectations is often used with a focus on adhering to the standard of care and promoting positive patient outcomes.

CLINICAL ISSUES

A common complaint of new nurses is their perceived lack of preparation regarding the various clinical skills. As an advanced beginner new nurses must master many skills in a relatively short time. Many of the skills are taught and practiced during nursing school, so you will want to continue to build on the foundation begun there. Practicing assessment skills on friends and family members is a great way to hone your skills, especially if it has taken you a long time to find your first position. Another idea is to volunteer to mentor undergraduate nursing students in the skills lab at your nursing school. This is a great way to polish your own skills and something you can add to your résumé. You can complete the skills checklist at the end of this chapter to help you develop a plan for review and practice. These are the most common ones you will be expected to complete when working on a medical–surgical unit. Some of the more advanced skills may not have been taught in nursing schools. For example, if you are assigned to an orthopedic floor you will most likely have to work with a continuous passive motion (CPM) machine, which is used for patients who undergo surgery for a total knee replacement (TKR). If you work in a specialty area, such as oncology, you will need to complete a course specific to the care of the oncology patient and the administration of chemotherapeutic agents. Some competencies are complex and require completion of a formal class, passing an exam, return demonstration, and observation.

Austin (2008) described seven key principles to promote patient safety and to protect you from a legal standpoint. The first principle is medication administration. Medication administration is a major responsibility of the hospital-based nurse, and you will spend a good portion of your shift administering medications to your patients. Medication administration requires using the nursing process, comprehensive knowledge of medications, diligence, and adherence to policies and procedures. Not only must you follow the "five rights" of medication administration, you must also know why your patient is receiving this medication and how it may interact with the other medications that have been ordered for the patient. You also need to evaluate the patient's response to the medication. For example, you administer an oral pain medication at 2 p.m. so you should reassess the patient at 3 p.m., or as per the hospital policy. Some hospitals have implemented a "quiet zone" during medication administration to help reduce errors due to distraction.

The next principle is to "monitor for and report deterioration." As a nurse you are expected to assess and reassess your patient throughout your shift, and to promptly follow up on any changes in patient status. Failure to do so may place the patient in danger and put you at risk of legal action.

The third principle is to "communicate effectively" with patients, families, nurses, and other members of the interprofessional team. The Joint Commission has specific guidelines regarding reporting when transferring patients. Using "SBAR" (situation, background, assessment, and recommendation) is a helpful tool when notifying the licensed health care provider about changes in patient condition.

The fourth principle is "delegate responsibly," which can be very challenging. Austin (2008) recommends checking with your state board of nursing for guidelines on delegating and following the "five rights" for delegating. "The "five rights" for delegating to another caregiver provide an easy-to-remember guide: right person, right task, right circumstance, right direction, and right supervision" (Austin, 2008, p. 37). In the hospital setting you will most likely be delegating tasks to unlicensed assistive personnel, and as the licensed person you are responsible for supervising them and knowing their scope of practice, in addition to the hospital's policy. For example, a nursing assistant may turn and position patients every 2 hours; however, the assistant cannot perform a pressure ulcer risk assessment. Furthermore, as the licensed nurse you must supervise the nursing assistant to be sure he or she is indeed performing the tasks that you have assigned.

The next principle is to "document in an accurate and timely manner" and follow your hospital's policy. The medical record is a legal document and is used to document care, and helps to ensure continuity of care by communicating with other members of the health care team (Austin, 2008).

The sixth principle is to "know and follow facility policies and procedures" which should reflect current nursing standards of care and practice, and as long as they are followed correctly will help to protect you from legal actions.

The last principle is to "use equipment properly." You should not use equipment unless you have been properly trained in its use and it is in perfect working order (Austin, 2008).

Providing holistic nursing care to your patients is a very serious responsibility and these seven principles can be used to inform your practice and help you to promote positive patient outcomes. Teamwork and collaboration, one of the QSEN (Quality & Safety Education for Nurses) competencies, is an essential in the delivery of holistic care. In recent years experts have realized how important it is to break down silos and work together to provide optimal care. Every single employee in a health care setting is vital to the success of the organization. Furthermore, the interprofessional team shares the common goal of providing evidenced-based holistic care that will promote positive patient outcomes.

Another vital component of patient care is the "shift-to-shift" report and unfortunately not all reports are equal. An exemplary report includes a brief overview of the patient's chief complaint and provides details about the patient's progress and current status in addition to the plan of care. Although policies vary across organizations walking rounds should be done as they provide an opportunity for direct observation and confirmation of patient status. For example, the night nurse states that the patient has a wound vac dressing, but when you go in the room it is not attached. At this point the problem can be addressed immediately; however, if you do not do walking rounds you may not discover this until the night nurse has left for the day. Furthermore, the patient will not be receiving the level of care he or she requires, which may result in liability. Learning how to give a good shift report takes time and practice. Nurses often use a report sheet, which can be very helpful because it guides the nurse as to the important topics to include. For example, patient's room and initials, medical dx (diagnosis), nursing dx, treatments, activity, diet, diagnostic tests, and special instructions. A good way to use your report sheet is to write the initial report that you receive in black ink, and then add your findings throughout the shift in red ink or pencil. This way you will be able to accurately share with the oncoming nurse the patient's history and the events that took place during your shift. It is also important to listen carefully to the report, take notes, and clarify any issues. Reports are also given when transferring patients to another unit, which may include both verbal and written communication. Once again, following your hospital's policies and procedures will be quite helpful when learning how to give and receive reports.

CULTURAL ISSUES

The health care arena is a complex and diverse setting with patients, families, and employees who have various cultural beliefs, practices, and values. "Providing culturally congruent care is a goal for which healthcare providers develop an individualized plan of care based on the patient's cultural values and beliefs" (Jeffreys, 2010;

Leininger, (1991); as cited in Hunt, 2014). Many nursing programs include a course on transcultural nursing or at the very least thread the concepts throughout the various nursing courses. Your organization will also provide some education on cultural diversity. Continuing to learn about different cultures and providing culturally congruent care will help you in your workplace. Culture may have a significant impact on health and wellness and nurses must be sensitive to the needs of their patients and families. Cultural beliefs are influenced by a person's ethnicity, religion, gender, and birthplace and include rituals, beliefs, and practices (Andrews & Boyle, 2008; Galanti, 2008; Hunt, 2013; Purnell, 2002). Although it is not possible to know all cultures, having a basic understanding of some of the predominant cultures in your geographic location is helpful (Hunt, 2012). Furthermore, many individuals migrate and over the years have developed their own subculture so never presume to believe a person will think, act, or feel based on their dominant culture. It is also helpful to complete a self-assessment of your cultural beliefs and values so that you can identify issues that require you to become more culturally sensitive (Andrews & Boyle, 2008). You may not agree with many of the practices, however, you are not there to judge so as long as no harm is done you need to figure out a way to come to terms with your beliefs. Oftentimes, health care providers do not understand the significance of a practice or belief. For example, a Jewish patient may be upset if he or she cannot light a Shabbat candle, or a Muslim patient may be upset if he or she cannot kneel on the prayer cloth to pray. Or a Catholic patient may be upset if someone mistakenly discards their scapula. If you are culturally sensitive you will facilitate, within reason, your patient's requests. Knowing that Latina families are very close and gather around the hospital bed of a family member who is ill should prompt you into developing a plan that will work for that patient and the other patients on the unit. Clearly, if a patient is in a double room it is not conducive to healing to have a bunch of people in one room, and it might violate health codes. However, developing a compromise in which the family can take turns visiting with the patient is a good solution.

Eye contact and touch are two other areas that are drastically different among cultures. For example, in the United States and many European countries eye contact is a sign of respect. Conversely, in the Asian and Muslim culture it is a sign of disrespect to make direct eye contact. Because touching is taboo in many cultures it is best to avoid it, except when providing direct care. Miscommunication is often at the heart of many misunderstandings so it is best to avoid jargon and gestures that may have different connotations across cultures (Andrews & Boyle, 2008; Galanti, 2008; Hunt, 2013; Jeffreys, 2010; Purnell & Paulanka, 2008). Many people believe in folk healing; some use a combination of modern medicine and folk healing. Using the four Cs of culture when assessing patients who practice folk medicine can be very helpful. The first "C" is "what do you call your problem?" (Galanti, 2008, as cited in Hunt, 2013). According to Galanti (2008), what modern medicine identifies as epilepsy is called "spirit catches you and you fall down" in the Hmong culture. One can see how this leads to a conflict in treating this disorder. The second "C" is "what do you think caused your problem?" If a person believes a spirit, or "mal ojo" also known as "the evil eye," instead of a bacteria or other physiological imbalance caused his or her illness, he or she will not believe that modern medicine can help. The third "C" is "how do you cope with your illness?" For example, did you visit a healer, perform a ritual, or take medicine? And the fourth "C" is "what are your concerns?" For example, do they think it is a serious issue or "are they worried about complications?" (Galanti, 2008). Certain health care remedies, such as "coining" and "cupping" may be misconstrued as a form of abuse. Both of these involve warming either a coin or cup and placing it on the affective area. These may leave red marks on a patient's skin but for the most part they are safe.

Hot and cold illnesses are common in the Latina and Asian cultures; certain illnesses are considered hot, and require cold drinks and foods, and vice versa. For example, pregnancy is a hot condition so hot foods and liquids should not be consumed (Galanti, 2008). Oftentimes, if an individual comes to the hospital he or she is seeking help from modern medicine, however, incorporating some of their folk beliefs can be very helpful. The following acronym may be used:

C: Care enough to learn about your patient's and family's cultural values, and beliefs.

A: Always complete a thorough cultural assessment of your patients and do your best to provide culturally congruent care.

R: Realize that many people develop their own unique culture, beliefs, and values.

E: Evaluate your own beliefs and try not to judge others for their cultural beliefs and practices (Hunt, 2014).

Not only will you be caring for a diverse group of patients, you will also be working with a diverse group of employees, thus it is important to be sensitive to your colleagues and their cultural beliefs.

PROFESSIONALISM

Professionalism is apparent in the way you dress, your conduct, your demeanor, and your communication skills. Nurses are socialized into the profession as students and continue to develop as professionals as they transition into practice and move through Benner's (1980) stages of novice to expert. As a registered professional nurse you will want to portray a professional image. Professionalism relates to a commitment to one's profession and the underlying tenets include education, research, community service, publications, membership in a professional organization, autonomy, competence, code of ethics, theory, and continuing education (Çelik & Hisar, 2012). These are the core components of professionalism. Celik and Hisar (2012) found that increasing levels of professionalism are related to job satisfaction. Depolitti (2008) found that it can take a nurse up to 3 years to develop a professional identity. According to McNamee (2013) nurses can demonstrate their professionalism by continuing their education and competency development. Communications, both written and verbal, are associated with professional behavior. Therefore, you will want to be sure you are using proper language and correct grammar, in addition to avoiding slang. Remember to address others by their surnames, unless they have advised you to call them by their first name or a nickname. Don't forget to provide your name and title on the phone, when meeting colleagues, and when entering a patient's room. The way a nurse dresses is associated with professionalism. Interestingly, Wocial et al. (2010) found that types of uniforms in the adult unit were related to professionalism; however, this was not true in the pediatric units. Perhaps this is due to the fact that pediatric nurses often wear colorful scrubs. All organizations have a dress-code policy with some selecting one uniform color for the entire organization, whereas others select colors according to specialty. The color of the uniform may be important to some; however, what is more important is being well groomed and neat in appearance. For example, this means a uniform that is clean and wrinkle free, polished shoes, long hair pulled back, minimal jewelry, and short manicured nails with light or no polish depending on dress code. Joining professional organizations and continuing one's formal and informal education helps one to develop her or his professional role.

PATIENT ADVOCACY

Patient advocacy is one of the most important roles of the registered nurse. "A patient advocate is someone who defends the patient against 'infringements of his or her rights" (Winslow, 1984, as cited in Mahlin, 2010).

The nurse advocate is defined as:

> the nurse is to actively support patients in speaking up for their rights and choices, in helping patients to clarify their decisions, in furthering their legitimate interests, and protecting their basic rights as persons, such as privacy and autonomy in decision making. (Hamrac, 2000, as cited in Mahlin, 2010)

Nurses are primary patient advocates because they spend a significant amount of time caring for their patients and families while developing holistic and therapeutic relationships. Nurses advocate for their patients/families in many ways. Patient advocacy includes helping patients with various aspects of their care such as teaching them about their diagnoses and discussing treatment options, providing information about community resources, and helping them to identify their own priorities (The Center for Patient Partnerships at the University of Wisconsin-Madison, 2014).

Providing patient-centered care is at the foundation of nursing advocacy and nurses ensure that patient's understand their plan of care. They also advocate for patients when they are giving informed consent for an invasive procedure. The nurse may not be obtaining informed consent as that is the role of the health care provider who is performing the procedure, however, he or she does verify that the patient understands the procedure and that he or she has the right to consent or not. Furthermore, if the patient is hesitant and needs further explanation the nurse will inform the surgeon, for example, and let the surgeon know he or she needs to come back and speak with the patient. The role of the advocate can be tenuous, and although nurses are not the only advocates they do spend the most amount of time with the patient. Nurses also protect the rights of patients by supporting the Patient Bill of Rights and autonomy of the patient. Promoting and protecting patient autonomy is one of the most important roles of a patient advocate. Patients have the right and freedom to self-determination. Nurses play a key role in supporting the patient's right to self-determination. The Patient Self-Determination Act was passed in December of 1991. "Federal Law requiring health care organizations who receive Medicare and Medicaid to provide written information to their patients regarding their right to make health care decisions" (Burkhardt & Nathaniel, 2002, p. 216). "Nurses play an important role as patient advocates in cancer care. The literature reviewed for this article showed that nurses use their role to promote and safeguard the well-being and interests of their patients" (Vaartio-Rajalin & Leino-Kilpi, 2011, p. 530). In summary, patient advocacy is a central responsibility and nurses must remember that the patient's wishes should be respected and his or her rights protected at all times.

PATIENT SAFETY, QUALITY OF CARE, AND PATIENT OUTCOMES

Patient safety and quality of care go hand in hand and nurses play an integral role in these two areas, although the entire health care team is responsible for quality of care and patient outcomes. Nurses must collaborate and coordinate care among the interprofessional team. Suhonen et al. (2012) found that individualized care is related to patient outcomes, such as patient satisfaction, which is also related to quality of care.

Patient satisfaction is a common goal shared by administrators and the interdisciplinary team. Patient satisfaction is related to decreased lengths of stay and most organizations are very concerned with their patient satisfaction scores. "The goal of the nurse is the patient's well-being, and this is realized through the interaction between them, an experience transpiring in whatever cultural context or healthcare setting in the world" (Tejero, 2012, p. 994). Nurses play a central role in addressing the needs of patients and families. Tejero (2012) found that nurse–patient dyads significantly impact patient satisfaction. Furthermore, they each play a role in patient satisfaction. Zane (2012) completed a review of the literature on caring and patient satisfaction and concluded that further studies are needed to measure this concept. One way to improve patient satisfaction is through the implementation of relationship-based care, which encompasses a philosophy that is patient centered and then builds evidence based on professional nursing practice. It does this by changing the way clinicians connect to patients, families, colleagues, physicians, and administration. The relationship-based care model was developed by Koloroutis (2004). "Relationship-based care is focused on a caring and healing environment which is vital to the quality of patient care" (Woolley et al., 2012, p. 179). This framework is patient centered and has three crucial relationships: relationship with patients, relationship with coworkers, and relationship with self (Koloroutis, 2004). Woolley et al. (2012) described the implementation of the relationship-based care model in the hospital setting. They posit that the implementation of this model was related to decreased falls, patient satisfaction, decrease in patient use of call bells, and decrease in hospital-acquired pressure ulcers. Relationship-based care places the patient at the center and requires nurses to deliver patient-centered care. Engaging in self-care in order to care for others is another component. Centering oneself prior to entering a patient's room, sitting at eye level and making eye contact are additional components of this model (Gibbons, 2012). Winsett and Hauck (2011) found that implementing a relationship-based care model was positively related to observable caring behaviors and nurse turnover. Patient outcomes and satisfaction levels also improved. Because of the positive effects of this model many organizations are beginning to embrace it and it is highly likely that you will work in an organization that has implemented relationship-based care.

SUMMARY

This chapter focused on your transition to your professional role, with an emphasis on clinical roles and competencies. The significance of the nursing process and prioritization were discussed and a template on "the 5-minute" assessment and self-assessment of common clinical skills were presented. Professionalism and patient advocacy were also presented, and an overview of cultural issues was given. The relationship of patient satisfaction, quality of care, and patient outcomes was discussed, and the relationship-based care model, which has been widely embraced by many health care organizations, was presented.

DISCUSSION QUESTIONS

1. Discuss the nursing process and its significance in your role as a nurse.
2. How can you improve your ability to prioritize care?
3. Explain how Maslow's hierarchy of needs can help you to prioritize care.
4. Why is clinical competency important?

5. Discuss the seven key principles identified by Austin (2008) to promote patient safety.
6. Describe the role of the patient advocate.
7. How does a patient's culture inform your practice?
8. What is professionalism?
9. Why is patient satisfaction important?
10. Discuss the relationship-based care model.

SUGGESTED LEARNING ACTIVITY

- Complete a self-assessment of clinical competencies.
- Complete an online self-assessment on cultural beliefs.
- Interview a nurse about her or his role as a patient advocate.
- Write an essay on the relationship-based care model.
- Practice your 5-minute assessment on friends or family members.

APPENDIX: FIVE-MINUTE ASSESSMENT: PERSON AND ENVIRONMENT

This is a guide to use for the initial assessment of your patient/patients.

Take six deep breaths before you enter the room to center yourself.

Wash your hands and don personal protective equipment (PPE) if required.

Introduce yourself to the patient (if culturally appropriate, make eye contact).

Verify patient identification as per policy.

Observe the patient and the environment for safety issues.

Assess the patient and the environment.

Follow a systematic pattern:

Take vital signs, including pain assessment.	
Head/neurology, LOC (loss of consciousness), responsiveness, orientation, pupils.	
Cardiovascular, chest pain, skin color, heart sounds, pulse, Intravenous (IV) fluids (verify IV orders), IV site.	
Respiratory,respiratory rate, color, O_2 saturation, breath sounds, use of oxygen (verify O_2 orders).	
Gastrointestinal system, bowel sounds (4 quadrants), abdominal assessment (soft, distended, tender, etc.),	
NPO (nothing per os), diet, presence of nasogastric tubes, drains, or dressings, enteral feeds (verify enteral feeds).	
Genitourinary system,urine output, bladder distension? Foley, urine color, consistency, etc.	
Lower extremities, pulse, edema, use of sequential compression devices (SCDs).	
Skin, turgor, intact, pressure ulcers, use of specialty mattresses.	
Be sure to check environment, equipment, and safety issues.	
Document findings.	
Report and follow up on any issues.	

CLINICAL SKILLS – SELF ASSESSMENT (PLEASE CHECK ANY SKILL THAT YOU FEEL YOU NEED TO PRACTICE)

_____Irrigation of GI (gastrointestinal) tubes, determination of tube placement

_____Administration of tube feeding through nasogastric, gastrostomy, and jejunostomy tubes

_____Female and male catheterization

_____Tracheostomy care and suctioning

_____Oral pharyngeal and nasopharyngeal suctioning

_____Discontinuing an IV

_____Administering PO (by mouth) or topical medications

_____Administering IM (intramuscular) medications

_____Administering SQ (subcutaneous) medications

_____Hanging IV tubing and bags

_____Assessment of and care of chest tubes

_____Assessment of and care of central lines

_____Central line dressing change

_____ Pressure ulcer care

_____Wound care

_____Drains (Jackson Pratt [JP], Hemovac)

_____ Sequential compression devices

_____ Care of ventilator patients

_____ Care of post operative patients

_____ Patient teaching

_____ Documentation

REFERENCES

Allen, D. (2013). Evidence shows staff ratios can work. *Nursing Standard, 27*(43), 20–22.

Austin, S. (2008). Safe nursing care. *Nursing, 38*(3), 35–39.

Benner, P. (1984). *From novice to expert: excellence and power in clinical nursing practice*. Menlo Park, CA:Addison-Wesley.

Burkhardt, M., & Nathaniel, A. (2002). *Ethics & issues in contemporary nursing* (2nd ed.). Clifton Park, NY: Delmar Thomson Learning.

Çelik, S., & Hisar, F. (2012). The influence of the professionalism behaviour of nurses working in health institutions on job satisfaction. *International Journal of Nursing Practice, 18*(2), 180–187. doi:10.1111/j.1440-172X.2012.02019.x

Center for Patient Partnerships, University of Wisconsin-Madison. (2014). *Overview of services*. Retrieved from http://www.patientpartnerships.org/advocacy/our-services/overview/

Clarke, K. (2004). Maslow: Hierarchy of needs—Or reflective framework? *N2N: Nurse2nurse, 4*(2), 27–28.

Deppoliti, D. (2008). Exploring how new registered nurses construct professional identity in hospital settings. *Journal of Continuing Education in Nursing, 39*(6), 255–262. doi:10.3928/00220124-20080601-03

Hunt, D. (2013). *The new nurse educator: Mastering academe*. New York, NY: Springer Publishing.

Hunt, D. (2014). Cultural competence in nursing practice: Gaining knowledge is the first step toward understanding. *ADVANCE for Nurses*. Retrieved from http://nursing.advanceweb.com/Continuing-Education/CE-Articles/Cultural-Competence-in-Nursing-Practice-2.aspx

Galanti, G. A. (2008). *Caring for patients from different cultures* (4th ed). Philadelphia: PA: University of Pennsylvania Press.

Gibbons, M. (2012). Relationship-based care: Respecting the sanctity of the patient room is the first lesson. *ADVANCE for Nurses*. Retrieved from http://nursing.advanceweb.com/Features/Articles/Relationship-Based-Care.aspx

Giger J., Davidhizar, R., Purnell, L., Harden. J., Phillips, J., & Strickland, O. (2007). American Academy of Nursing Expert Panel report: Developing cultural competence to eliminate health disparities in ethnic minorities and other vulnerable populations. *Jornal of Transcultural Nursing, 18*(2), 95–102.

Jannings, W., Underwood, E., Almer, M., & Luxford, B. (2010). How useful is the expert practitioner role of the clinical nurse consultant to the generalist community nurse? *Australian Journal of Advanced Nursing, 28*(2), 33–40.

Jeffreys, M. (2010). Overview of key issues and concerns and dynamics of diversity: Becoming better health care providers through cultural competence. In *Teaching cultural competence in nursing and health care* (2nd ed., pp. 3–44). New York, NY: Springer Publishing.

Koloroutis, M. (2004). *Relationship-based care: A model for transforming practice.* Minneapolis, MN: Creative Healthcare Management.

Leininger, M. M. (1991). Culture care diversity and universality theory and evolution of the ethnonursing method. In M. M. Leininger (Ed.), *Culture care diversity and universality: A theory of nursing.* (pp. 1–42). New York: National League of Nursing Press.

Lubbe, J., & Roets, L. (2014). Nurses' scope of practice and the implication for quality nursing care. *Journal of Nursing Scholarship, 46*(1), 58–64. doi:10.1111/jnu.12058

Mahlin, M. (2010). Individual patient advocacy, collective responsibility and activism within professional nursing associations. *Nursing Ethics, 17*(2) 247–254.

Maslow, A. H. (1943). A theory of human motivation. *Psychological Review, 50*(4), 370–396.

Maslow, A. H. (1954). *Motivation and personality.* New York, NY: Harper and Row.

McLeod, S. A. (2007). *Maslow's hierarchy of needs.* Retrieved from http://www.simplypsychology.org/maslow.html

McNamee, M. (2013). How do RNs demonstrate to the public that we are professionals? *Canadian Nurse, 109*(8), 19.

Purnell, L. (2002). The Purnell model for cultural competence. *Journal of Transcultural Nursing, 13*(3), 193–196.

Purnell, L. D., & Paulanka, B. J. (2008). *Transcultural health care: A culturally competent approach* (3rd ed.). Phildelphia, PA: F.A. Davis.

Shekelle, P. (2013). Nurse-patient ratios as a patient safety strategy: A systematic review. *Annals of Internal Medicine, 158*(5 Pt. 2), 404–409. doi:10.7326/ 0003-4819-158-5-201303051-00007

Suhonen, R., Papastavrou, E., Efstathiou, G., Tsangari, H., Jarosova, D., Leino-Kilpi, H., & … Merkouris, A. (2012). Patient satisfaction as an outcome of individualised nursing care. *Scandinavian Journal of Caring Sciences, 26*(2), 372–380. doi:10.1111/j.1471-6712.2011.00943.x

Tejero, S. (2012). The mediating role of the nurse-patient dyad bonding in bringing about patient satisfaction. *Journal of Advanced Nursing, 68*(5), 994–1002. doi:10.1111/j.1365-2648.2011.05795.x

Theisen, J. L., & Sandau, K. E. (2013). Competency of new graduate nurses: A review of their weaknesses and strategies for success. *Journal of Continuing Education in Nursing, 44*(9), 406–414. doi:10.3928/00220124-20130617-38

Vaartio-Rajalin, H., & Leino-Kilpi, H. (2011). Nurses as patient advocates in oncology care. *Clinical Journal of Oncology Nursing, 15*(5), 526–532. doi:10.1188/11.CJON.526–532

Winsett, R. P., & Hauck, S. (2011). Implementing relationship-based care. *Journal of NursingAdministration, 41*(6), 285–290. doi:10.1097/NNA.0b013e31821c4787

Wocial, L., Albert, N., Fettes, S., Birch, S., Howey, K., Jie, N., & Trochelman, K. (2010). Impact of pediatric nurses' uniforms on perceptions of nurse professionalism. *Pediatric Nursing, 36*(6), 320–326.

Woolley, J., Perkins, R., Laird, P., Palmer, J., Schitter, M., Tarter, K., & Woolsey, M. (2012). Relationship-based care: Implementing a caring, healing environment. *MEDSURG Nursing, 21*(3), 179–184.

Zane Robinson, W. (2012). Systematic review of effect of a caring protocol provided by nursing staff on patient satisfaction of adult hospitalized patients. *International Journal For Human Caring, 16*(4), 58–70.

CHAPTER 12

Delegation

The secret of success is not in doing your own work but in recognizing the right [person] to do it.

—Andrew Carnegie

Never leave that till tomorrow which you can do today.

—Benjamin Franklin

OBJECTIVES

At the end of this chapter the reader will be able to:

- Describe the art of delegation
- Understand importance of delegation and supervision
- Describe strategies for delegation
- Identify tasks that may be delegated

Delegation is one of the most difficult skills nurses, especially new nurses, have to master. Although delegation may be taught in nursing school there is little time to practice this skill. Furthermore, Henderson et al. (2006) found that only 41% of nurses had been taught about delegation in nursing school. Delegation is extremely important and must not be taken lightly as patient safety is at stake. Many nurses believe that delegation is something for higher level nursing leaders, however, this is an erroneous assumption, although nursing leaders are required to delegate on a larger scale (Nies, 2011). Because nursing units are comprised of a skill mix (RNs [registered nurses], LPNs [licensed practical nurses], PCTs [patient care technicians], and NAs [nursing assistants]) nurses are required to delegate and supervise the other patient care providers. Learning the art of delegation will help you to develop your skills and become competent in this role. The current National Council Licensure Examination (NCLEX-RN®) test plan also includes many questions relating to delegation because it is so integral to the role of the nurse (Henderson et al., 2006). Delegation involves much more than assigning a task for a subordinate and improper delegation may place a patient at risk. "The process of delegating requires the RN to remain accountable for the task. However, the delegated individual also assumes responsibility for the task and answers to the RN" (Saccomano & Pinto-Zipp, 2011, p. 523.) Saccomano and Pinto-Zipp (2011) found that associate degree nurses and diploma school nurses find delegation more challenging than baccalaureate nurses, but after 5 years they are all at the same level. They also found that education and experience were directly related to competence in delegation. However, leadership style, which was a variable in their study, was not related to competence in delegation. This chapter focuses on understanding delegation and how to delegate in a safe and effective manner.

ART OF DELEGATION

The art of delegation relates to learning how to delegate in a manner that is professional and respectful, fair, and consistent in addition to being based on scope of practice of the staff members. A general definition of delegation is "Grant of authority by one party (the delegator) to another (the delegatee) for agreed purpose(s). Under the legal concept of vicarious liability, the delegator remains responsible for the delegate's acts or omissions in carrying out the purpose of the delegation" (BusinessDictionary.com, 2014). According to a joint position statement by the American Nurses Association (ANA) and the National Council of State Boards of Nursing (NCSBN, 2005), delegation is an important skill for nurses to master and if done correctly can promote safe and effective patient care. Furthermore, nurses should seek advice from their mentors and follow the hospital's policies and procedures, standards of care, and their state's practice act. "The strength of an organization comes from the diversity, not the conformity, of its skills and capabilities. An organization is a team of individuals with unique gifts, backgrounds, personalities and strengths" (Nies, 2011, p. 6). Each individual adds to the richness of the patient care environment and everyone has a valuable role to play. It is important to recognize this when you are delegating. Being on a health care team is similar to being in an orchestra, where all the musicians must play their parts under the direction of the conductor. If one person does not play his or her part correctly the song will not sound good. If the conductor gives the wrong directions to the musicians the music will be off key. Furthermore, the conductor is responsible for overseeing the orchestra. As the registered professional nurse your role will be similar to the role of the conductor. You will have to give directions as needed at the right time to the appropriate person. The art of delegation also involves being respectful and cognizant of the person's role, knowledge, and capabilities. Although the staff member may have no choice but to follow your directions, you do not want to be abrasive or authoritarian. Remember the old adage, "you get more flies with honey than vinegar." Everyone has the right to be treated in a respectful manner. Treating others how you would like to be treated is another suggestion. As a staff nurse, and in the future, as perhaps a nurse manager, you will be both the delegator and delegatee, which will help you to appreciate the art of delegation. One must also be reasonable and realistic when delegating. If you delegate too many tasks to a person she or he will feel overwhelmed and at best will complete some of the tasks, or at worst nothing will be completed. Consider for a moment an 8-ounce glass, which can only hold 8 ounces of liquid. If you try to put in 10 or 12 ounces it will overflow. Ultimately, you are responsible for the work that you delegate so be mindful of this as you are delegating tasks. If you are new to delegating this will certainly take time for you to grasp, however, during your orientation you observed your preceptor so let that be your guide. Part of your overall goals for the day must include a plan for how you will delegate and how you will monitor and ensure that the required tasks are completed in a safe and effective manner. The relationship you develop with your colleagues is important, and you want to foster team spirit because you need to work together in harmony and do not want to create an adversarial work environment. In summary, the art of delegation requires knowledge, competence, courage, and compassion.

DELEGATION ACTIVITIES

Delegation is something that all nurses must learn how to do. It is not an easy task, however, one must develop strategies to do this so patient care will never be jeopardized. One hopes you have been taught about delegation as a student. You should also be educated about delegation during your orientation. Furthermore, you will have many opportunities to observe your preceptor delegating throughout the day. It is important to pay close attention to this so that you can learn how to do this while you are on your own. Prior to delegating you must be well versed in your hospital's policies and procedures, state board regulations, and scope of practice. You also need to take into account the acuity of the patient because some patients may be too complex for unlicensed assistive personnel (UAP; Haslauer & Jones, 2003). When a patient has a high acuity level and requires a high level of care it is best to work with the UAP when providing care. Following your hospital policies and procedures is of the utmost importance because although your state board may allow for delegation your organization may not support all the tasks that would be allowed in accordance with the scope of practice and the state boards of nursing. For example, although feeding patients is often within the scope of practice of a nursing assistant, your organization may not support this practice due to potential aspiration. Or it may have a specific policy that the patient's swallowing and gag reflex be assessed by a speech pathologist prior to assigning an unlicensed assistive person to feed a patient. Each organization has different policies so always verify the policy prior to taking any action.

The board of nursing or regulatory agency in your state or country may also have specific guidelines regarding delegation of tasks. Be sure to visit the site and look up the information. As a rule it is better to look things up and verify for yourself instead of relying on another person because he or she may have incorrect information. This caveat applies to everything; it is always best to go to the primary source because you are responsible for your own actions both as a student and a nurse.

The National Council of State Boards of Nursing (2014) provides definitions for the various nursing roles, which may be helpful in understanding the various licensed, certified, and unlicensed roles within the health care system. A registered nurse (RN) is licensed by the state board of nursing after passing the NCLEX_RN® exam. A licensed practical nurse (LPN) must pass the NCLEX-RN exam and works under the supervision of a registered nurse. An advanced practice registered nurse (APRN) is an RN who has completed an advanced degree program and can diagnose and prescribe in accordance with state guidelines. A certified nursing assistant (CNA) provides direct patient care under the supervision of the RN. A UAP is unlicensed and performs tasks under the supervision of the RN.

All state boards of nursing have scope-of-practice statements for registered nurses and licensed practical nurses, however, only some state boards have scope-of-practice statements for nursing assistants. For example, in New Hampshire the following scope-of-practice statement can be found online.

SCOPE OF PRACTICE (RN AND LPN)

326-B:12 Scope of Practice; Registered Nurse:

I. An RN shall, with or without compensation or personal profit, practice nursing that incorporates caring for all clients in all settings, is guided by nursing standards consistent with standards established by the National Council of State Boards of Nursing and approved by the board, and shall be limited to:

  (a) Providing comprehensive nursing assessment of the health status of clients, families, groups, and communities.

  (b) Collaborating with a health care team to develop an integrated client-centered plan of health care.

  (c) Developing a plan of nursing strategies to be integrated within the client-centered health care plan that establishes nursing diagnoses, setting goals to meet identified health care needs, prescribing nursing interventions, and implementing nursing care through the execution of independent nursing strategies and prescribed medical regimen.

  (d) Delegating and assigning nursing interventions to implement the plan of care.

  (e) Providing for the maintenance of safe and effective nursing care rendered directly or indirectly.

  (f) Promoting a safe and therapeutic environment.

  (g) Providing health teaching and counseling to promote, attain, and maintain the optimum health level of clients, families, groups, and communities.

  (h) Advocating for clients, families, groups, and communities by attaining and maintaining what is in the best interest of the client or group.

  (i) Evaluating responses to interventions and the effectiveness of the plan of care.

  (j) Communicating and collaborating with other health care professionals in the management of health care and the implementation of the total health care regimen within and across care settings.

  (k) Acquiring and applying critical new knowledge and technologies to the practice of nursing.

  (l) Managing, supervising, and evaluating the practice of nursing.

  (m) Teaching the theory and practice of nursing.

(n) Participating in the development of policies, procedures, and systems to support the client.

(o) Other nursing services that require education and training prescribed by the board and in conformance with national nursing standards. Additional nursing services shall be commensurate with the RN's experience, continuing education, and demonstrated competencies.

New Hampshire also requires that their nursing assistants be licensed.

SCOPE OF PRACTICE; LICENSED NURSING ASSISTANT

I. An LNA shall, with or without compensation or personal profit, practice under the supervision of an RN, APRN, or LPN.

II. An LNA is responsible for competency in the nursing assistant curriculum approved by the board. LNAs are authorized to administer medication when they hold a currently valid certificate of medication administration and under the circumstances established by the board through rules adopted pursuant to RSA 541-A.

III. Following successful completion of the curriculum, a nursing assistant shall be able to:

(a) Form a relationship, communicate, and interact effectively with individuals and groups.

(b) Demonstrate comprehension related to individuals' emotional, mental, physical, and social health needs through skillful, direct nursing-related activities.

(c) Assist individuals to attain and maintain functional independence in a home or health care facility.

(d) Exhibit behaviors supporting and promoting care recipients' rights.

(e) Demonstrate observational and documenting skills required for reporting of people's health, safety, welfare, physical and mental condition, and general well-being.

(f) Provide safe nursing-related activities under the supervision of an RN or an LPN (New Hampshire State Board of Nursing, 2014).

There is also a specific scope of practice for licensed practical/vocational nurses and although this may vary among states and countries it is important to know that they cannot assess, so you need to consider this when delegating. For example, if you have a new admission they can do the vital signs and history but cannot complete the required assessment.

Working on a nursing unit is a team effort and everyone must know his or her roles and responsibilities so you will not have to be constantly delegating, however, you do need to make sure that the required tasks are completed. Each person is also responsible for his or her own actions. Most of your delegation will relate to additional tasks that may be required. For example, you may need the nurse assistant to take another set of vital signs or obtain a urine sample. You might need the LPN to administer a stat medication. Or you might need the patient care technician to do a simple dressing change on a patient. Keep in mind you will still have to assess the wound, but if dressing changes were in the scope of practice of the technician he or she could change the dressing. The goal is to ensure quality of care and positive patient outcomes.

Another resource when learning about delegation is to review the job descriptions of the various roles. This will help you to learn about the specific roles and responsibilities of the various staff members at your organization. Some organizations have these available online, or they may be in a policy book on the unit. You should be provided with a copy of your job description during orientation. This is an extremely important document and you should read it very carefully. The job description can also be helpful if someone does not feel she or he should be asked to complete a particular task. An easy way to settle this type of conflict is to review the job description together. If a staff member refuses to complete a task that is within his or her scope of practice and in accordance with his or her job description and hospital policy you will need to report this to your immediate supervisor.

Some of the common tasks you may delegate to a nursing assistant are activities of daily living (ADLs) such as bathing, grooming, and feeding; vital signs (temperature, pulse, and respirations); turning and positioning; ambulation; and obtaining certain specimens. Technicians have a broader scope of practice and can usually take blood pressures and blood glucose measurements, and do simple dressing changes. LPNs have a much broader scope and can administer most medications (although in some locations they cannot administer the first dose of an intravenous antibiotic), administer various treatments, and document care. Teamwork and collaboration should be done in a way that motivates the UAP, helps the nurse to improve delegation skills, and promotes positive patient outcomes (Saccomano & Pinto-Zipp, 2011). Saying "please" and "thank you" and recognizing the person's efforts and accomplishments will also be very helpful.

STRATEGIES FOR DELEGATIONS

The way you delegate is the key to successful delegation. According to Haslauer and Jones (2003), "The delegation process consists of five steps: assessment, planning, accountability, supervision and evaluation" (p. 23). Prior to delegation you must assess the situation, the patient, the UAP, and the task you are planning to delegate. Planning involves how you will approach and delegate. Using communication skills is very important as you want to be very clear and direct. Accountability relates to your role as the delegator and your responsibility to ensure that the delgatee completed their assignment. Furthermore, you must continue to assess your patients. Ongoing evaluation of patient outcomes and the competence of the assistant must be completed. If the employee does not complete the assigned task, or does not do it correctly, you should consult with your supervisor (Haslauer & Jones, 2003). Using your communication skills is foundational to successful delegation. Being sure to communicate respectfully and clearly are extremely important (Potter et al., 2010). It is helpful to meet with your team at the beginning of the shift and develop a plan for the day. You want to be sure to communicate to your nursing assistants that you are a team and share the goal of meeting the needs of the patients. Building team spirit creates a positive work environment and will most likely result in improved patient outcomes. Working with your team members is also very helpful. Nursing assistants will appreciate the fact that you are working with them. Furthermore, many of them have years of experience and insights into the needs of the patient. Some nurses do not recognize the important role the UAPs play in promoting patient outcomes, which results in conflict. "The National Council of State Boards of Nursing (1995) in the United States has identified five rights of delegation: right task, right circumstances, right person, right direction or communication and right supervision" (Potter et al., 2010, p. 161). Following these five rights can be very helpful when learning how to delegate. The right task relates to scope of practice. For example, you cannot delegate medication administration to your UAP. The right circumstances can relate to the type of patient, or the acuity of the patient. The right person is making sure you select the correct person to whom to delegate the task. For example, you may ask the unit secretary to bring a specimen to the lab (if that is part of the job description); however you could not delegate vital signs to the secretary. The right direction requires clear instructions as to what needs to be completed. This should include the patient, the room number, the specific task or tasks, the time and frequency of the task, and the follow-up. The right supervision requires you to verify that the tasks have been completed and that they have been done correctly. For example, you assign the UAP to take stat vital signs and to bring you the results. If the UAP reports vital signs that are extremely different from the previous set of vital signs you need to go and double check the vital signs yourself. Or if the UAP does not report back to you in a few minutes you would need to investigate why. Of course, you would need to take care of the patient first and then you would have to address this with the UAP. Depending on the circumstances there may be a reason why the UAP did not follow your directions. However, if he or she clearly disregarded your directions you will need to consult with your manager because this type of behavior is unacceptable and places the patient at risk of harm. Ultimately you are responsible, so if something happens to the patient you will be liable. Potter et al. (2010) described the conflicts that occur between the registered nurses and the nursing assistive personnel (NAP) regarding delegation such as role conflict and work ethic. Age played a factor in conflicts especially with young RNs and older NAPs. Work ethic was another issue, with both the NAPs and the RNs viewing each other as not working hard enough. Role conflict presents another issue, with the NAPs questioning why they were being asked to do tasks that the RNs could do. The RNs were frustrated when the NAPs did not want to do a certain task. Personality was a factor and many RNs found that NAPs would outright refuse to do certain tasks. On a positive note, Potter et al. (2010) did find that communication, teamwork, and collaboration did lead to successful delegation. Clearly, there needs to be ongoing education and development in addition to support from nursing education and leadership. Following the strategies that were outlined above will be very helpful as you learn how to delegate.

BARRIERS TO EFFECTIVE DELEGATION

There are many barriers to effective delegation, which include factors related to the delegator and the delegatee. One major barrier for a new nurse is lack of confidence and being intimidated by NAPs/UAPs who are older and have worked in the unit for many years. They may question the authority of the new nurse and test him or her to see how the new nurse is going to react. Although it may be hard to stand up to someone you must be guided by the fact that you are the licensed person and patient advocate. If you avoid delegation you will quickly burn out as you will not be able to keep up with all the work and will begin to feel frustrated and overwhelmed. You will also put your patient at risk. The key is to develop a good relationship with your colleagues. If you are respectful and fair in your delegation most of the staff will respond positively. You also don't want to delegate because you think something is beneath you. For example, you just administered medications to your patient and the patient asks for the bedpan. Unless you need to give a stat med to another patient you can probably offer the bedpan to the patient instead of asking the NAP to help the patient. If you have to finish administering medications you can let the NAP know that you placed the patient on the bedpan and you would like the NAP to check on the patient. You do not want the NAPs to resent you because then they will become resistant, so be mindful of the necessity of your delegation.

Another barrier relates to lack of trust in the NAP's abilities (Curtis & Nicholl, 2004). You may not believe the NAP is going to do the task in the correct manner so you avoid delegating. If you do not believe the NAP is capable of doing a task that falls under her or his responsibilities, then you should notify your nurse manager. Every employee is expected to be able to perform all the duties outlined in his or her job description and if unable to do so, he or she may need further education and training. This should be communicated to your manager and you can also instruct the staff in a positive way.

Workload may also be a barrier to successful delegation. If there are not enough staff to care for the patients everyone is going to become overwhelmed and stressed. This may lead to over delegation, which will have a negative effect on the staff and the patients. You will not always have an adequate amount of staff, but you need to resist the temptation to place the extra burden on the NAPs. You can always ask your mentor, preceptor, or nurse manager for guidance when figuring out how to delegate.

Lack of knowledge regarding each other's roles and responsibilities is another factor. Oftentimes the RNs believe they are busier than the NAs and conversely, the NAs believe they are busier than the RNs. Although they are both busy, the NAP may not fully appreciate the nurse's roles and responsibilities, in addition to the process of medication administration and the critical thinking and time the RN needs to administer medications to a group of patients (Potter et al., 2010). Holding team meetings to openly discuss these issues can be very helpful.

Another issue that may hinder the delegation process is over- or underdelegating (Henderson et al., 2006). If you overdelegate you actually increase the risk of adverse events as the NAP/UAP will not be able to do everything and may not have the critical-thinking skills to prioritize care. For example, Mr. S requests clean bed linen because there are crumbs in his bed, and Mrs. T needs to be turned and repositioned every 2 hours. If the NAP/UAP feels overwhelmed he or she may decide to complete only one task. Clearly the turning and repositioning are a priority; however, the NAP/UAP may decide to change the linen instead because Mr. S has rung the bell four times in the past 30 minutes. If you under delegate you may also place patients at risk because you may not be able to complete all the tasks that need to be done. Although you may be able to do this for a short time eventually you will become stressed, which may lead to job dissatisfaction and burnout. Finding a balance is difficult but with time you will figure out what is a fair amount of delegation. Think about your own experiences and how you might feel if your supervisor gave you way too many tasks to complete. You would probably feel overwhelmed, annoyed, and frustrated. Being empathetic to the needs of your team members and supporting them is very important and will benefit everyone. Staffing issues can also place a barrier on delegation (Henderson et al., 2006). When there are not enough staff on the unit it causes everyone to feel overwhelmed and stressed. Sometimes you are caught between a rock and a hard place because there is no easy way to complete all the tasks that need to be done. When this happens, you should consult with your manager and work with the team members to develop a plan to prioritize care and maintain patient safety and positive patient outcomes.

In summary, learning the art of delegation and addressing potential barriers takes time, however, due to the complexity of patients' needs, registered nurses must learn how to delegate effectively.

CRUCIAL CONVERSATIONS AND DELEGATION

Communication is foundational to being an effective delegator. Using the principles of therapeutic communication is very helpful. Patterson et al. (2012) described crucial conversations and how following the eight principles of "crucial conversations" can be helpful when dealing with difficult situations.

For example, it is important to identify the issue and then figure out what you want to accomplish. Next you need to deal with your stress and be respectful and nonthreatening. It is important to think about what you want to say, try to be persuasive, and consider alternative solutions (Patterson et al., 2012).

These principles can be used in many different situations, for example, when dealing with difficult people, when asking for a raise, or when dealing with sensitive issues. These principles can help you to develop exemplary delegation skills.

ROLE PLAYING: SCENARIO 1

Role playing can be very helpful when developing delegation skills. You can do this with your friends, family members, or fellow nurses. Develop a list of tasks that you would delegate and take turns being the registered nurse and the NAP/UAP. Think about different scenarios and situations and how you might improve the process. Develop situations based on the content of this chapter. For example, a new nurse needs to delegate tasks to a nursing assistant who is older and has been employed for 30 years. The new nurse is intimidated and unsure as to how to approach the nursing assistant. When she finally does approach the nursing assistant, the nursing assistant is rude and ignores the request. What should the new nurse do? Should she self-evaluate her actions and see if a different approach would have been better? Was the delegation within the scope of practice? Should she try again or should she consult with the manager? How might the eight principles of "crucial conversations" be used in this type of situation?

SCENARIO 2: INAPPROPRIATE REQUEST

In this scenario you are the delegatee and the doctor is the delegator. The doctor is new and is evaluating a patient who is having cardiac issues. He tells you to administer IV (intravenous) Digoxin 0.25mg IV stat. However, you know that in your organization RNs are not allowed to push IV Lanoxin (Digoxin). You try to explain this to the doctor but he gets angry and tells you he will report you if you do not administer the medication. He also says you are putting the patient at risk. What would you do? Would you give the medication because the doctor ordered it? Would you explain to him that it is not in your scope of practice and that you can get the vial of Digoxin and needle but he will need to administer it? Would you speak to your manager? This is a case of the doctor not knowing the scope of practice of the nurse. Clearly, you cannot administer this medication and if the doctor refuses to do it himself you would need to report the situation to your nurse manager.

SCENARIO 3: DELEGATION TO AN NAP

In this scenario you are a new nurse and need to delegate to your nursing assistant. She is older and has worked on the unit for 20 years. At the beginning of the shift you met with the nursing assistant and discussed the plan for the day. She offered suggestions based on her experience and you found them helpful. You used the five steps of delegation and everything worked fine. The nursing assistant and you worked together as a team and you both completed your patient assignments. The patients were safe and satisfied. And the nurse manager complimented you both for doing such a great job.

There are positive and negative situations related to delegation. Using all the recommendations will improve the delegation process, although at times you may encounter a very difficult person and need the assistance of your preceptor and manager.

TOP 10 TIPS FOR SUCCESSFUL DELEGATION

1. Use the "five rights" of delegation.
2. Read the scope of practice and board of nursing regulations on delegation.
3. Know your hospital's policies and procedures.
4. Foster teamwork and collaboration.
5. Know your job description and the job descriptions of the delegatees.
6. Use communication skills.
7. Be fair and balanced when delegating.
8. Use the key principles of "crucial conversations."
9. Consult with your preceptor and manager for guidance on delegating.
10. Remember that you are accountable and must evaluate the patient and the delegatee.

SUMMARY

This chapter focused on the art of delegation and the importance of using delegation strategies. Delegation is an important skill for nurses to master and there are strategies that one can employ to improve delegation skills. Delegation must be based on scope of practice, policies and procedures, and board of nursing guidelines. One must also consider the skill set of the delegatee and remember that he or she is ultimately accountable and must verify that the tasks were done correctly and that patient safety was maintained and patient outcomes were positive. It takes time and experience to learn how to delegate and eventually you will master this skill.

DISCUSSION QUESTIONS

1. Discuss the salient points of the art of delegation.
2. What factors guide the nurse when delegating?
3. What are the "five rights" of delegation?
4. Identify and describe three strategies for delegation.
5. What are some barriers to delegation?
6. What are the eight key principles of "crucial conversations"?
7. What steps might you take if a person refused to comply with your delegation?
8. What would you do if someone delegated something to you that was beyond your scope of practice?
9. How might you foster teamwork and collaboration with your colleagues?
10. What are the negative effects of underdelegation and overdelegation?

SUGGESTED LEARNING ACTIVITIES

- Role play a delegation scenario.
- Read the scope of practice on your board of nursing's website.
- Interview a nurse and nurse manager about delegation.
- Interview an NAP/UAP about his or her views on delegation.
- Read three current articles on delegation.

REFERENCES

Ales, B. (1995). Mastering the art of delegation. *Nursing Management, 26*(8), 32A.

American Nurses Association. (2005). *Joint ANA and National Council of State Boards of Nursing position statement*. Retrieved from https://www.ana.com

Businessdictionary.com (2014). *Delegation*. Retrieved from http://www.businessdictionary.com/definition/Delegation.html#ixzz2wzTN0fxh

Curtis, E., & Nicholl, H. (2004). Delegation: A key function to nursing. *Nursing Management, 11*(4), 26.

Grenny, J. (2009). Crucial conversations: The most potent force for eliminating disruptive behavior. *Physician Executive, 35*(6), 30–33.

Haslauer, S., & Jones, D. (2003). Delegation—Concept, art, skill, process. Article adapted with permission from the Arkansas Nursing News. *ASBN Update, 7*(1), 22–24.

Henderson, D., Sealover, P., Sharrer, V., Fusner, S., Jones, S., Sweet, S., & Blake, T. (2006). Nursing EDGE: Evaluating delegation guidelines in education. *International Journal of Nursing Education Scholarship, 3*(1), 1–10.

Kærnested, B., & Bragadóttir, H. (2012). Delegation of registered nurses revisited: Attitudes towards delegation and preparedness to delegate effectively. *Nordic Journal of Nursing Research & Clinical Studies / Vård I Norden, 32*(1), 10–15.

National Council of State Boards of Nursing. (2014). *Definitions of nursing roles*. Retrieved from: http://www.ncsbn.com.

New Hampshire State Board of Nursing. (2014). *Scope of practice: Licensed nursing assistant*. Retrieved from http://www.nh.gov/nursing

Nies, T. (2011). The art of delegation. *Smart Business Cincinnati/Northern Kentucky, 7*(6), 6.

Patterson K., Grenny, J., McMillan, R., & Swizler, J. (2012). *Crucial conversations: Tools for talking when stakes are high* (2nd ed.). New York, NY: McGraw-Hill.

Potter, P., Deshields, T., & Kuhrik, M. (2010). Delegation practices between registered nurses and nursing assistive personnel. *Journal of Nursing Management, 18*(2), 157–165. doi:10.1111/j.1365-2834.2010.01062.x

Saccomano, S. J., & Pinto-Zipp, G. (2011). Registered nurse leadership style and confidence in delegation. *Journal of Nursing Management, 19*(4), 522–533. doi:10.1111/j.1365-2834.2010.01189.x

CHAPTER 13

Leadership Development

If your actions inspire others to dream more, learn more, do more and become more, you are a leader.

—John Quincy Adams

OBJECTIVES

At the end of this chapter the reader will be able to:

- Describe key leadership theories
- Describe leadership styles
- Identify the various leadership roles in nursing
- Discuss the relationship between emotional intelligence and leadership styles
- Describe the Institute of Medicine's *Future of Nursing* report and leadership
- Develop a plan for continued development as a nursing leader

There are many different roles required of the nurse and leadership is integral to all nurses. Granted there are different levels of leadership, however, every nurse must possess leadership qualities, which can be cultivated as nurses progress in their careers. Registered professional nurses are expected to serve as team leaders and eventually charge nurses on their units. They may also be asked to chair hospital-wide committees. One of the key recommendations of The Institute of Medicine's report *The Future of Nursing* calls for nurses to be prepared to assume key leadership positions in various health care sectors to lead change and advance health (Robert Wood Johnson Foundation, 2010).

Some individuals are born to lead and this role comes quite easily to them, however, most individuals need to develop their leadership skills. Learning about the various leadership theories and styles will help you to develop your own style and to plan for a future leadership position.

LEADERSHIP THEORIES

There are a plethora of leadership theories, including the seminal "great man" theory and, more recently, transformation leadership. Historically, the belief was that leaders were born not made and that certain males were born with leadership qualities, hence the "great man" label (Bolden et al., 2003). Today the belief is that leaders may be born with inherent leadership traits but that they need further development to be successful and exemplary leaders (Hunt, 2012). The "great man" theory can be credited to Thomas Carlyle (1841), who described how great men shaped history through their leadership, inspiration, and their intellect. "In the 1930s, numerous leadership trait studies were conducted and from these a list of traits of an effective leader was identified. These included intelligence, task-relevant knowledge, dominance, and self-confidence, and energy, tolerance for stress, integrity, and emotional maturity" (Hunt, 2012, p. 55).

Trait theories examined whether an individual possessed leadership traits before or after becoming a leader. Eventually this led to the development of the behaviorist theories. The behaviorist theories posit that leaders are made not born and that anyone can develop the skills needed to be a good leader. Behaviorist leaders embrace an *initiation* structure—leaders make sure their employees get the job done—or a *consideration* structure—a leader respects and values his subordinates (George & Jones, 2005). Situational leaders base their style of leadership according to the situation and their style may vary from participative, which is more laissez faire, to autocratic, which is more dictatorial (Bolden et al., 2003). The *leader/member exchange theory* (Graen & Uhl-Bien, 1995) identifies dyads between the leader and the individual instead of the leader and the group (Lunenberg, 2010). There are two types of dyads: the "in" group and the "out" group. It is certainly more desirable to be a part of the "in" group, as these members participate in decision making. Conversely, the "out" group members are closely supervised doing the work they are contractually hired to do (Lunenberg, 2010).

The transactional leader is directive and influential and serves as a figure of authority. Subordinates are expected to follow orders and there is a clear chain of command. The transactional leader believes people are motivated by rewards and punishments and need clear directions to do a good job (Giltinane, 2013). One of the newer widely embraced theories is that of the transformational leader. The transformational leader is charismatic and is one of the most desirable types of leaders, especially in nursing and in Magnet hospitals. Transformational leaders help subordinates realize their full potential and influence them to consider what is best for the organization instead of their personal needs (Bolden et al., 2003; George & Jones, 2005; Giltinane, 2013). Green (2005) posits that the most effective leaders are transformation because they encourage rather than coerce.

Bass and Avolino(1994) described the four I's of Transformational Leadership:

- **Idealized influence (charisma)**
  - admired and respected by followers
  - shares risk
  - considers followers' needs
  - behaves ethically and morally (trustworthy)
- **Inspirational motivation**
  - gives meaning and challenge to work
- **Intellectual stimulation**
  - uses creative problem solving
- **Individualized consideration**
  - listens, praises

These types of leaders are respected because they are morally and ethically bound and support subordinates. They also collaborate with them to reach goals. Kouzes and Posner (2007) have studied leadership for many years and have developed a leadership model. In their model they describe the behaviors of an exemplary leader. The behaviors are: model the way, inspire a shared vision, challenge the process, enable others to act, and encourage the heart. Their model describes an exemplary and transformational leader who inspires others through role modeling and support. They have also developed a tool to measure the behaviors of leaders that is based on these five practices. There is a version for self and a version for subordinates to complete; this instrument has been widely used in multiple research studies (Hunt, 2012).

LEADERSHIP STYLES

Kurt Lewin (1939) described several leadership styles based on his research. These styles were autocratic, democratic, and laissez-faire (Goleman, 2000). Leaders develop different styles based on their inherent traits, personal beliefs, experiences, role models, mentors, and education. Furthermore, they may need to change their style based on the situation and/or the subordinate. The *authoritative leader* may be described as bossy or dictatorial. However, because an authoritative leader provides a clear vision and direction this is one of the most effective styles, especially when there is little time for collaboration, such as in an emergency situation. Most subordinates do not like this type of leadership style. The *democratic* leader participates with the subordinates as both a leader and a team member, seeks input from the group, and engages the group members in meeting goals and expectations. The third style is the *affiliative*; these leaders aim to promote harmony and can be helpful in improving the morale of the employees (Goleman, 2000). The least effective style is *laissez-faire* because with this method the leader lets the subordinates do what they want and offers little or no guidance.

Kerfoot (2013) describes the relationship of fatigue and leadership style and posits that many nursing leaders, because of the way they are taught, are more authoritarian and controlling. She further states that leadership based on micromanaging may lead to fatigue. Therefore, nurse leaders need to be taught how to be transformational or participatory leaders. According to Kerfoot (2013) the key to effective leadership involves:

- Surrounding yourself with the right people
- Creating structures in the work environment to develop effective employees
- Doing the work of the leader and letting the staff do their own work

Empowering subordinates and serving more as a transformational leader is often the most effective style of leadership. One must change his or her belief that no one can do the work as well as he or she can. Therefore, exemplary leaders must also know how to be effective delegators (see Chapter 12). Whether you are serving as a team leader, nurse manager, or vice president for nursing you need to understand theories and styles in addition to the positive and negative aspects of the various styles.

IOM *FUTURE OF NURSING REPORT* (LEADERSHIP)

In 2008, the Robert Wood Johnson Foundation (RWJF) and the Institute of Medicine (IOM) launched a 2-year initiative to respond to the need to assess and transform the nursing profession. A committee was formed and a blue print for the future of nursing was created. The report, *The Future of Nursing: Leading Change, Advancing Health*, was published in 2010. The report has four key messages and eight recommendations. The seventh recommendation is to "prepare and enable nurses to lead change to advance health" (RWJF, 2010). According to the report nursing leaders and educators need to prepare the nursing workforce to assume leadership positions across all levels and in private and public organizations. Currently action coalitions across the country are developing and implementing programs to achieve this recommendation (Bleich, 2013). The report calls for nurses to lead the way in advancing health care (Wyatt, 2013).

Clearly, we have our work cut out for us as nurses make up less than 3% of community health system boards, compared with approximately 20% who are physicians (IOM Summit, 2013). Another factor in accomplishing this recommendation relates to entry-into-practice requirements and the lack of leadership development in associate degree and diploma programs. Furthermore, although baccalaureate-prepared nurses are provided with the foundational leadership theory and clinical experiences, they require additional development and education to become exemplary leaders. Even nurses prepared at the master's and doctoral level will most likely require further leadership development, especially if they want to be considered for a position on a health system board. Strech and Wyatt (2013) suggest that nurses be full partners in policy and collaborate on health care redesign. It is time for nurses to assume their leadership roles and take their rightful place at the policy table.

EMOTIONAL INTELLIGENCE

Emotional intelligence (EI) has become an important concept in the world of nursing leadership. "The concept of EI was introduced and defined in 1990 by Peter Salovey and Jack Mayer. It was further popularized in 1995 with the publication of the book 'Emotional Intelligence' [*sic*] by Daniel Goleman, a science reporter and psychologist" (Feather, 2009, p. 376).

"Emotional intelligence relates to non-cognitive skills and has been associated with the ability to become successful in one's life. Indeed, successful individuals need to have both emotional intelligence and cognitive intelligence" (Freshwater & Stickley, 2004, as cited in Hunt, 2013). Emotional intelligence relates to one's ability to be aware of emotions of self and others. It also relates to the ability to use emotions positively to develop judgments and employ emotional knowledge. Another aspect is having the ability to consciously regulate your emotions (Feather, 2009). Although there is a paucity of evidence in regard to emotional intelligence and the role of the nurse leader, there are studies that demonstrate the positive effects of developing emotional intelligence. "According to Caruso et al. (2002), using emotions allows leaders to understand and motivate others through expression of multiple perspectives that can enable planning and engagement of employees in activities" (as cited in Feather, 2009, p. 379). A leader may be very intelligent; however, without emotional intelligence the leader may let emotions cloud the issue.

EXEMPLAR

Mary Smith is a new nurse on a medical–surgical unit. She just completed her 6 months of orientation and is now working independently. Her nurse manager has her master's degree and 3 years of leadership experience. Mary is nervous because this is her first day on her own and the unit is very busy. She voices her concerns to the nurse manager. The nurse manager is very overwhelmed at this point and tells Mary to stop whining and get to work. Mary is shocked that the nurse manager would speak to her in this manner and becomes more anxious. She confides in her mentor who spends some time speaking to Mary and gives her some guidance and support. Her mentor also shares that this behavior is very common in this nurse manager and although the nurses have tried to talk to her she becomes very defensive. The staff nurses have requested a meeting with the administration to discuss this pervasive issue.

If this nurse manager had developed emotional intelligence, she most likely would have been able to control her emotions and spend a few minutes reassuring Mary. Granted, even people with high levels of emotional intelligence may have a bad day once in a while and react in a negative way. However, this manager's actions are not reflective of EI.

Many experts believe that emotional intelligence can be developed through formal education and training programs. However, some experts do not see the validity of emotional intelligence. Sadri (2012) described the results of her review on emotional intelligence and concluded that many leadership development programs include at least some of the competencies developed by Goleman, which include self-awareness, self-regulation, motivation, empathy, and social skills. Sadri (2012) recommends that organizations teach each skill independently to help leaders develop. Clearly there seems to be some merit to the emotional intelligence model, and because of the paucity of research studies in measuring emotional intelligence and conflicting reports further investigation is warranted.

MENTORS AND LEADERSHIP ROLE

The benefits of mentoring have been discussed previously in this book; however, due to the significant role mentors play in leadership development it is worth discussing mentors further, especially in regard to leadership (Pate, 2011). Mentors come in and out of lives at different points in time and serve different purposes. For example, one might have an academic mentor, then a professional mentor. Although a mentor can guide you in many different areas, when it comes to developing as a leader you need a mentor who is an exemplary leader. You need a mentor who will "model the way" (Kouzes & Posner, 2007) because this person will influence the type of leader you become. And in turn you will become a leader who will model the way. According to Kouzes and Posner (2014), leaders set an example for others and help them develop interim goals and achieve victories. This is what you need to look for in your mentor, but how will you know whether they are an exemplary leader or not? Clearly, you will need to do some research on your potential mentor. You might consider nurse managers, clinical directors, or charge nurses. It depends on the type of role you are striving to obtain. For example, if you are interested in becoming a charge nurse, then you might select a mentor who is an experienced charge nurse. On the other hand if your goal is to become a nurse manager, then you will want to select an experienced and exemplary nurse manager. One way to decide is to observe the manager and make discreet inquiries about his or her leadership styles and background. For example, what is his or her level of education? Has she or he completed formal leadership development training? Is he or she a supportive leader? Does he or she possess the five practices of an exemplary leader? Kouzes and Posner (2014) have developed a tool called the Leadership Practices Inventory; there are two versions, one for the leader to self-evaluate and one for the staff nurse to evaluate the nurse manager. You can obtain a copy of the instrument and review the items to see whether the nurse manager exhibits those qualities.

Kelly and Hagerman (2013) described a program in their organization that was focused on developing emerging nurse leaders (ENLs). The program was based on Kouzes and Posner's (2007) five practices of exemplary leadership and used a mentor/mentee model. Formal classes were offered and required that the mentors be experienced nurse leaders and that the mentees have 5 years of experience, a desire to develop professional leadership, and the intention of remaining in the profession for at least 10 more years. The mentors and mentees attended four training sessions and the mentees developed a project. The results were positive with the mentees feeling empowered and realizing that with support they could affect positive changes. "The program also highlighted for them the personal and professional growth that can occur during a mentoring relationship" (Kelly & Hagerman, 2013, p. 28). Although the results were positive there were some negative issues, such as organizational barriers, and challenges of finding time to connect with each other (Kelly & Hagerman, 2013). Vann (2014) described the relationship of the Institute of Medicine's report *The Future of Nursing* (2010) and mentoring and posits that "Mentoring supports the third key message by encouraging leadership development and collaboration" (p. 16). Furthermore, "leadership is cultivated through effective mentoring" (Vann, 2014, p. 16). Hill et al. (2005) investigated the relationship of mentoring and leadership development in African American women and found that it played a role in personal and professional development. McCloughen et al. (2009) described mentoring and the developmental stages the mentor and protégé progress through as they develop their reciprocal mentoring relationship (Vance, 2010). McCloughen et al. (2009) found that mentors unconditionally champion the careers of their mentees, and that mentees possessed a leadership vision (p. 326). They also indicated that the first theme to emerge in their study was the connection between the mentor and mentee. Three subthemes also emerged: *considering each other with positive regard, developing respectful boundaries,* and *honoring key human characteristics* (p. 329). Clearly developing a mutual respect for each other was integral to this relationship and an important point to keep in mind when collaborating with a mentor.

Remember, when you develop a relationship with a mentor it is a two-way street: You both need to work together. Vance (2010) describes the mentor connection as a reciprocal relationship. Whether you engage in a formal or informal process for selecting your mentor you will need to develop goals, guidelines, and boundaries. Before you invite someone to be your mentor think about what you are hoping to gain/give from/to this relationship.

ASSESSMENT OF LEADERSHIP STYLE

There are many tools available online for you to assess your leadership style. This type of activity can be very helpful when developing your plan for a future leadership role.

SELF-DEVELOPMENT OF LEADERSHIP SKILLS

Leadership development begins when you are born and continues throughout your life. Some leadership qualities are inherent and others are learned or acquired. Some well-known traits of leaders include:

- Intelligence
- Task-relevant knowledge
- Dominance
- Self-confidence
- Energy
- Tolerance for stress
- Integrity
- Emotional maturity
- Emotional intelligence
- Empathy
- Caring
- Knowledge
- Fairness
- Excellent communication skills
- Charisma and ability to inspire

Consider the list of traits and whether or not you possess them. How might you develop or improve on these traits? Completing a self-assessment of your leadership style is the first step in your formal development. You may complete Kouzes and Posner's (2007) Leadership Practices Inventory for self-assessment, which you will find on their website: www.lpi.com. Then you can use this information to create a plan for development. Seeking out leadership roles is another important step. You might volunteer to lead a support group or journal club at your place of employment. Becoming a charge nurse is a great way to function as a leader with the support of your nurse manager. Think about how you would like your manager/leader to treat you and treat others in that manner. Being a leader can be stressful so be sure to use the strategies on self-care that were discussed in Chapter 3.

Depending on the type of leadership position you are aspiring to, you may need to continue your education. Educational development should include formal academic programs, continuing education classes, and informal on-the-job training. Be sure to take advantage of any programs that are available to you. Most midlevel nursing leadership positions require a master's degree, although some organizations will hire experienced bacca-laureate nurses who have leadership potential and agree to return to school to earn an advanced degree. Aduddell and Dorman (2010) described the benefits of a value-added education for graduate level nursing curriculum.

Therefore, you want to carefully select the academic program when you are advancing your education. If you know you want to be a nursing leader you may want to select an administrative track, or at least a combined program that offers courses in leadership development.

As stated above, finding a mentor who is an exemplary leader is highly recommended. Role playing is another great way to develop your leadership skills. Using the principles of communication and crucial conversations can also be very helpful when serving as a leader (see Chapter 12). Leaders need to be fair, for example, if you are the charge nurse and developing the patient assignment for the day you need to consider many factors, such as census, acuity, staffing mix, and competency. You also need to create a fair assignment for each individual that is based on these factors. Naturally, you may be closer to certain people on your unit, but you cannot "play favorites." There will always be some people who are unhappy with their assignments; however, you need to have confidence in your ability to stand by your decisions as long as they are sound ethical decisions that are grounded in fairness and made with caring and empathy. Pate (2011) recommends that ambulatory care nurses "adopt a strategy for themselves that emphasizes certain "core values" such as courage, honor, respect, and commitment" (p. 13), and suggests the following strategies for organizations to adopt for nurse leader education:

- Establish a networking group
- Offer education courses
- Start a journal club
- Start a shadowing program
- Foster a mentoring process
- Use AACN (American Association of Colleges of Nurses) core curriculum for ambulatory care nursing in continuing education
- Develop a clinical ladder

Although the author focused on ambulatory care nurses these strategies are applicable to all nursing specialties. All nurses should incorporate the "core values" into their daily practice because positive relationships and attributes will have a positive impact on patient outcomes, patient satisfaction, and nurse satisfaction.

In summary, all nurses possess leadership qualities that serve as the foundation for becoming an exemplary transformational leader. There are many leadership roles available to nurses and the only way to discover whether a leadership role is for you is to "test the waters" and experience the role. Sometimes, you may not see the qualities within yourself; however, your mentor or manager may and invite you to consider a leadership role. As a rule when opportunity knocks you should open the door and at least consider the opportunity.

FUTURE LEADERSHIP ROLES

There are many leadership roles in nursing and it is never too early to start planning and developing goals for achieving a leadership role. Certainly you will have an opportunity to observe your preceptor serving as team leader and eventually you will lead your team during your shift. Becoming a charge nurse usually requires at least 1 year of experience, however, if you show strong leadership abilities your nurse manager may begin to mentor you as a future charge nurse. The charge nurse is responsible for overseeing and managing the unit during a particular shift and reports directly to the nurse manager. Midlevel nurse manager roles and assistant manager roles are the next step in becoming a leader and require more experience and education. Each organization has different requirements so be sure to check with your manager or Human Resources Department. If this is a role you aspire to, then be sure to do everything in your power to develop your leadership abilities. Nursing supervisors, clinical directors, and assistant directors are other roles and require a master's degree and experience. These positions oversee the midlevel managers and require oversight of several units and many more employees. There are also clinical coordinator roles in many departments and specialties. The chief nursing officer or vice president for nursing is one of the highest levels and requires at least 10 years of leadership experience and a master's degree, with many organizations requiring a doctoral degree. This role is very challenging and comes with major responsibilities for overseeing the entire organization, nursing staff, and other departments. There are many other leadership opportunities, such as committee chairs, professional organizations (usually requires a vote), academic leadership roles, and on various health system boards. You might also serve as a leader in a community organization or civic group. Another way to serve as a leader is in the political arena, which certainly would benefit by have more experienced nurse leaders to influence health policy and workforce development. This is just an overview on potential leadership roles and if you desire to obtain one of these roles you should develop an action plan (see Table 13.1) as soon as possible.

Develop a list of objectives with a plan and objectives to meet your goal. Try to be realistic and develop measurable objectives.

TABLE 13.1
Action Plan Template

Goal: To obtain a leadership position in: _____				
Objectives	Plan	Due Date	Completed Y= yes N= no	Revised Plan

Top 10 Leadership Tips

1. Complete a self-assessment of leadership skills.
2. Continue your education.
3. Develop your emotional intelligence.
4. Find a mentor.
5. Develop a plan for obtaining a leadership role.
6. Always be fair and empathetic.
7. Respect others.
8. Be a good listener and communicator.
9. Seek guidance and support from your superiors.
10. Believe in yourself.

Summary

This chapter focused on leadership theories and styles and the need for nurses to assume leadership roles. The importance of self-evaluation and development as an exemplary leader was discussed. The relationship of emotional intelligence and leadership was reviewed in addition to the significance of the role of the mentor. Strategies for leadership development were reviewed and a brief overview of potential leadership roles was included.

DISCUSSION QUESTIONS

1. Discuss the "great man" theory.
2. List five leadership traits and discuss whether you possess them.
3. Describe the leader/member exchange theory.
4. What are the attributes of a transformational leader?
5. What are the five practices of an exemplary leader according to Kouzes and Posner (2007)?
6. List and describe the four styles of leadership and situations in which they are required.
7. List and describe three strategies for leadership development.
8. Discuss potential leadership roles.
9. What are the four "core values" of leaders and followers?
10. Identify one nurse leader who is a role model to you.

SUGGESTED LEARNING ACTIVITY

- Complete a self-assessment on leadership styles.
- Interview a nurse manager and a clinical director of nursing.
- Read three peer-reviewed articles on leadership and nursing.
- Develop a plan for obtaining a mid level leadership position.
- Role play scenarios with your peers and family members.
- Research Magnet hospitals, visit one, and interview a nurse leader.

REFERENCES

Aduddell, K., & Dorman, G. (2010). The development of the next generation of nurse leaders. *Journal of Nursing Education, 49*(3), 168–171. doi:10.3928/01484834-20090916-08

Bass, B. M. (1990). *Bass & Stogdill's handbook of leadership: Theory, Research, and Managerial Applications.* (3rd ed.). New York, NY: Macmillan.

Bass, B. M., & Avolio, B. J. (1994). *Improving organizational effectiveness through transformational leadership.* Thousand Oaks, CA: Sage.

Bass, B. M., & Bass, R. (2008). *The Bass handbook of leadership: Theory, research, and managerial applications.* (4th ed.). New York, NY: Free Press.

Bleich, M. R. (2013). The Institute of Medicine report on the future of nursing: A transformational blueprint. *AORN Journal, 98*(3), 214–217. doi:10.1016/j.aorn.2013.07.008

Bolden, R., Gosling, J., Marturano, A., & Dennison, P. (2003). A review of leadership theory and competency frameworks. *Centre for Leadership Studies.* Retrieved from http://www.leadershipstudies.com/documents/mgmt_standards.pdf

Carlyle, T. (1841). *On heroes, hero worship and the heroic in history.* Boston, MA: Adams.

Caruso D., Mayer J., & Salovey P. (2002). Emotional intelligence and emotional leadership. In R. E. Riggio & S. E. Murph (Eds.), Multiple intelligences and leadership (pp. 55–73). Mahway, NJ: Lawrence Erlbaum.

Feather, R. (2009). Emotional intelligence in relation to nursing leadership: Does it matter?. *Journal of Nursing Management, 17*(3), 376–382. doi:10.1111/j.1365-2834.2008.00931.x

Freshwater, D., & Stickley, T. (2004). The heart of the art: Emotional intelligence in nurse education. *Nursing Inquiry, 11*(2), 91–98.

George. J., & Jones, G. (2005). *Understanding and managing organizational behavior* (4th ed.). Upper Saddle River, NJ: Pearson-Prentice Hall.

George, J. M., & Jones, G. R. (2008). *Understanding and managing organizational behavior* (5th ed.). Upper Saddle River, NJ: Prentice Hall.

Giltinane, C. (2013). Leadership styles and theories. *Nursing Standard, 27*(41), 35–39.

Goleman, D. (2000, March/April). Leadership that gets results. *Harvard Business Review,* 78–88.

Graen, G. B., & Uhl-Bien, M. (1995). Relationship-based approach to leadership: Development of the leader-member exchange (LMX) theory of leadership over 25 years. *Leadership Quarterly, 6,* 219–247

Green, R. (2005). *Practicing the art of leadership* (2nd ed.). Upper Saddle River, NJ: Pearson-Prentice Hall.

Hill, J., Del Favero, M., & Ropers-Huilman, B. (2005). The role of mentoring in developing African American nurse leaders. *Research & Theory for Nursing Practice, 19*(4), 341–356.

Kelly, M., & Hagerman, L. (2013). Growing tomorrow's leaders. *Canadian Nurse, 109*(5), 26–29.

Kerfoot, K. M. (2013). Are you tired? Overcoming leadership styles that create leader fatigue. *Nursing Economic$, 31*(3), 146–151.

Kouzes J., & Posner, B. (2008). *The leadership challenge* (4th ed., pp. 3–26). San Francisco: John Wiley & Sons.

Lewin, K., Lippit, R., & White, R.K. (1939). Patterns of aggressive behavior in experimentally created social climates. *Journal of Social Psychology, 10,* 271–301.

Lunenberg, F. (2010). Member exchange theory: Another perspective on the leadership process. *International Journal of Management, Business, and Administration, 13*(1), 1–5.

McCloughen, A., O'Brien, L., & Jackson, D. (2009). Esteemed connection: Creating a mentoring relationship for nurse leadership. *Nursing Inquiry, 16*(4), 326–336. doi:10.1111/j.1440-1800.2009.00451.x

Pate, J. M. (2011). Educating and mentoring nurse leaders. *AAACN Viewpoint, 33*(4), 13.

Robert Wood Johnson Foundation Initiative on the Future of Nursing. (2010). *The future of nursing: Leading change, advancing health.* Retrieved from www.thefutureofnursing.org.

Sadri, G. (2012). Emotional intelligence and leadership development. *Public Personnel Management, 41*(3), 535–548.

Strech, S., & Wyatt, D. A. (2013). Partnering to lead change: Nurses' role in the redesign of health care. *AORN Journal, 98*(3), 260–266. doi:10.1016/j.aorn.2013.07.006

Vann, K. (2012). Mentoring: Creating tomorrow's nurse leaders today. *Nursing News, 36*(4), 16–17.

Wyatt, D. A. (2013). The future of nursing: Understanding who nurses are. *AORN Journal, 98*(3), 267–272. doi:10.1016/j.aorn.2013.07.012

Chapter 14

Issues and Solutions in Your New Role

The ultimate measure of a man is not where he stands in moments of comfort and convenience, but where he stands at times of challenge and controversy.

—Martin Luther King, Jr.

Objectives

At the end of this chapter the reader will be able to:

- Identify potential issues and challenges faced by new nurses
- Use strategies for overcoming challenges
- Understand the importance of time management and organizational skills
- Understand reality shock, burnout, job dissatisfaction
- Understand the importance of support and confidence
- Identify strategies to ameliorate issues with preceptors

There are myriad issues faced by new-graduate nurses; some are positive and unfortunately some are negative. Some of the topics in this chapter have previously been discussed in Chapter 10, however, that was in relation to the initial transition and this chapter focuses more on the period when you are completing your formal orientation and becoming more independent in your role. At this point you may still have the support of a preceptor, although many of you will be on your own with an informal network of support from the more experienced nurses on your unit. If your preceptor experience was not positive you may not feel prepared for this independent role. This may lead to reality shock, burnout, and job dissatisfaction in addition to lack of confidence. Taking a proactive approach instead of a reactive approach will help you to address the many issues faced by new nurses.

ISSUES WITH TIME MANAGEMENT AND ORGANIZATIONAL SKILLS

The significance of time management and organization, especially when you are working independently, cannot be ignored because the stakes are high when you are dealing with human lives. As you leave the comfort and support of your preceptor you will need to continue to improve your time management and organizational skills. Please refer back to Chapter 10 for strategies on time management and organizational skills. Although it is okay to spend some time socializing with your colleagues you need to be careful not to waste time, especially at the beginning of your shift, because once you fall behind in your assignment you will find it very difficult to get back on track. When this happens you may become stressed and also place your patients at risk as there will be a delay in assessment and interventions. A delay in assessment may result in a patient decompensating because you did not identify that the patient was unstable. A delay in treatment, such as administering a medication or nebulizer treatment, can also result in adverse outcomes. Be sure to verify the organization's policy on medication administration as many of them allow for an hour before and after the administration time as you will most likely be administering medications to a group of patients. Keep in mind that stat medication must be administered right away as soon as the medication is available. If there is a delay in treatment that is beyond your control you should document this and also consult with the charge nurse and/or nurse manager. You also need to provide your nursing assistant with a report and review the assignment and this must be done in a timely manner. Always be proactive and advocate for your patients and use your time wisely. Developing a plan at the beginning of your shift will help you to stay organized and manage your time effectively. Granted, some days are more hectic than others so it is vital to seek support if you are feeling overwhelmed. Even if you are no longer being precepted you can still consult with your preceptor, manager, or fellow staff nurses on your unit.

One particular challenge in regard to time management occurs when patients and families require more attention. This may be due to the complexity of their care or their need to receive moral support and information. One must be very savvy in managing time spent with patients and families. On the one hand you want to spend quality time with your patients, but on the other hand you have many tasks to accomplish. Time must also be spent with the interprofessional team to collaborate and discuss each patient's plan of care (Thylefors, 2012). Finding a balance is challenging; however, with time and experience you will discover a way to manage. Another challenge occurs when a patient becomes unstable and requires more nursing care. Using prioritization skills will certainly help, however, if one patient is very unstable you should seek support from your colleagues and/or manager/supervisor. Oftentimes nurses hesitate to seek help because they do not want to show they are vulnerable. However, patient safety is your biggest priority. Delegation may help but you can only delegate certain tasks to your nursing assistant, and what you may need is for the charge nurse/manager to change your assignment or request additional staff. Never be afraid to ask for help when you need it, but don't take advantage of your coworkers. Most nurses will empathize with you and lend a helping hand, unless they feel you are goofing off and wasting time. Be sure to do your best to manage your time effectively, realizing that some things are beyond your control. For example, if the night shift is disorganized and you receive a late report this may have a negative effect on how you organize your day. Furthermore, if you do not receive a comprehensive report you will need to spend more time reviewing the medical records so you have a better understanding of your patients' needs. It is to be hoped that you will work on a unit with a nurse manager who has exemplary leadership skills, which sets the tone for a well-organized unit.

EXAMPLE OF HOW YOU MIGHT ORGANIZE YOUR MORNING

6:40 a.m.—Arrive on unit and store belongings

6:55 a.m.—Check your assignment

7:00 a.m.—Receive report

7:20 a.m.—Organize your COW (computer on wheels) and restock drawers

7:30 a.m.—Assess your patients and document findings

8:00 a.m.—Give report to nursing assistant

8:15 a.m.—Review medical records and verify orders

8:30 a.m.—Administer 8 a.m. medications if ordered
8:45 a.m.—Check that patients have had breakfast
9:00 a.m.—Finish documenting if necessary and begin to administer
        10 a.m. medications
10:00 a.m.—Assist nurse assistant if needed and complete treatments
        such as dressing changes
10:30 a.m.—Attend interprofessional rounds
11:00 a.m.—Continue documentation
11:30 a.m.—Patient education
12:00 p.m.—Assist patients as needed

Keep in mind this is a guide that may need to be revised based on norms and policies of your unit, patients' condition, new admissions, discharges, and patients who need to be prepared for diagnostic tests or procedures.

According to Thomack (2012) time management requires goal setting, planning, and outcome measurement. It also requires balance and purpose. One must also be cognizant of how much time each task will require. Being organized relates to time management. Before you begin your day organize your COW or medication cart and stock your drawers. Think about what you will need to complete your tasks. Be sure to have your stethoscope, watch, pens, notebook, and any additional equipment. Stock your draws with alcohol wipes, tape, IV (intravenous) tubing, and IV flushes (as long as it can be locked and this is within your organization's guidelines). Consider approximately how much time you will spend with each patient. For example, if Mrs. Z is receiving medications via a nasogastric tube and has two IV antibiotics it will take longer to administer her medications compared to Mr. C, who is only scheduled to receive two oral medications. Of course, Mr. C may be unstable when you go to administer his medications and you may end up spending more time with him than Mrs. Z, therefore, the more organized you are the smoother your day will be. Cohen (2005) described time management in regard to nurse managers; however, many of the principles apply to staff nurses too. She suggests that the following items are considered time stealers for nurse managers:

- opting not to delegate
- allowing constant interruptions
- not knowing how to say, "No, I won't be able to; I'm already committed"
- planning poorly
- refusing to confront and address unacceptable employee behavior (Cohen, 2005).

Addressing these issues will be helpful to managers and staff nurses. We have already discussed the importance of effective delegation. Constant interruptions are not only time stealers they distract you and may cause you to make an error. In fact some hospitals have designated medication administration a time when nurses should not be interrupted unless it is an emergency. Learning how to say "no" to an extra assignment or obligation can be difficult; however, you don't want to get overwhelmed. Sometimes, the "new kid on the block" is assigned all the committee's work because the other nurses have been doing it for such a long time. Planning poorly is related to lack of organization and time management. The last item certainly is a bigger issue for nurse managers; however, you may experience this when you delegate tasks. If you do not confront a person who is refusing to complete his or her work you will not be able to complete all of your tasks in a timely manner. Although these items seem simple and are based on common sense, many individuals have difficulty addressing these issues. Interestingly, Lundgren and Segesten (2001) investigated nurses' use of time in a medical–surgical unit with an all-registered-nurse (RN) staff and found that over time nurses discovered a more coherent way of organizing tasks. This is based on the primary care model. However, most organizations use a skill mix when staffing their medical units. Primary care models are often used in a specialty unit, such as the intensive care unit. Every organization is different and you need to be flexible when working in different settings and environments.

REALITY SHOCK, ROLE STRESS, BURNOUT, AND JOB DISSATISFACTION

The literature is replete with studies on reality shock, role stress, burnout, and job dissatisfaction, which are all related to turnover (Lampe et al., 2011; Watts et al., 2013). Although these issues may affect all nurses, the numbers of new nurses who experience these problems are staggering, with Kovner reporting new-nurse turnover between 50% and 70% (2007). Reality shock was previously discussed and is something new nurses may experience when transitioning to their new roles and discovering that the real world of nursing is somewhat different than the ideological one of nursing school (Duchscher, 2009).

Burnout has been described as feelings that result in emotional exhaustion and decreased personal accomplishment. Nurses who are burned out may have difficulty sleeping, experience gastrointestinal issues, and headaches. Burnout may result in decreased satisfaction of patients and nurses, according to Watts et al. (2013), who found that organizational culture is related to burnout, and that making small changes (such as developing an innovative and challenging subculture) can fight it. New nurses often feel disillusionment, moral distress, and performance distress during the first few months of transition (Duchscher, 2009) and this may lead to burnout and job dissatisfaction.

Job satisfaction has been written about extensively in the literature and relates to how a nurse perceives his or her role and work environment. There are many factors that influence job satisfaction, such as support, autonomy, work environment, and physician–nurse collaboration (Coomber & Barriball, 2007; Utriainen & Kyngas 2009) Lynn, Morgan, and Moore (2009) define job satisfaction as "the extent to which a nurse is satisfied with his or her workload and the colleagues with whom he or she works" (p. 9). Beecroft, Dorey, and Wenton (2008) suggest that meeting new nurses' needs during orientation will result in increased job satisfaction and nurses who are competent practitioners. Knowing that these issues exist can help you to take a proactive approach and avoid some of these stressful situations. If you are feeling overwhelmed and stressed you need to advocate for yourself. Reality shock can be avoided if you prepare yourself for your role. Completing an externship, internship, working as a nursing assistant, or volunteering can help you to understand the difference between your supervised clinical rotations and the real world. Engaging in self-care and being a self-advocate are also recommended. Communicating with your preceptor, manager, and colleagues and letting them know how you are feeling can also be helpful. Journaling, which is discussed in Chapter 16, is a wonderful way to deal with the stress and anxiety of a new position. Taking a proactive approach also involves increasing your knowledge and reading the literature on these topics so that you can be prepared to face the many challenges that will arise. Sometimes we set the bar too high and become distressed when we are not "perfect," thus reading Benner's (1984) *Novice to Expert* can help you to set realistic goals for your journey into the world of nursing. Your knowledge and foundation must be solid so you can continue to build on them, much like the building of a house. If the house does not have a strong foundation it may not last very long. The Institute of Medicine's report *The Future of Nursing* (2010) calls for nurses to become lifelong learners. Clearly, nursing school cannot provide all the knowledge and experience you will require to be a proficient nurse, so one must be prepared to continue his or her formal and informal education. Possessing a solid knowledge base will serve you well—especially with medications. For example, as a nursing student you are expected to look up medications before administration and possibly write up drug cards—this is intended to prevent errors and to help you learn about the various medications. If you have to look up every medication as a registered nurse it will take you twice as long as it would if you have a strong knowledge base of the medications. This premise holds true for your assessment skills, clinical skills, medical conditions, treatments, and laboratory results. There is nothing wrong with looking things up to clarify, but when faced with something unfamiliar, however, being prepared will make a big difference. Continuing to learn and practice will help you to feel more confident and able to manage complex patients independently.

Some things are beyond your control and if you experience feelings of dissatisfaction or signs of burnout you need to critically analyze the situation. Perhaps the work environment is toxic and no matter how well prepared you are, you may not make a difference (Clare & Van Loon, 2003). Therefore, you may need to consult with the staff development educator and manager and perhaps a different unit will be the best option. Sometimes you have to make the decision to find a position in another organization that offers a more supportive work environment (Laschinger, Finegan, & Wilk, 2009). The person–environment (P–E) fit theory can help you to understand the relationship between the employee and the organization. "The basic tenets of P–E fit focus on a shared value between an organization and an employee. In some cases it is described as a reciprocal relationship of "needs" and "rewards" or whether the employee can meet the expectations of the organization" (Edwards, 2008, as cited in Hunt, 2012, p. 34). Therefore, if your needs are not being met by the organization or you are not meeting the needs of the organization the best option may be to search for a new position.

Leadership support is also an important factor in new-nurse job satisfaction. Hunt (2012) found that leadership support, especially from the nurse manager, was related to nurse job satisfaction. Although there are many excellent nurse managers, there are also nurse managers who are overwhelmed with their role and are not able to offer the level of support new nurses require. One hopes you will not experience any of these negative issues; however, if they do occur don't be too quick to blame yourself as there are many other factors. The most important thing is to recognize issues and take a proactive approach.

INADEQUATE ORIENTATION

The orientation program plays a major role in your success so be sure to make the most of it. Orientations that are not adequate in length or are not high in quality may result in lack of support and lack of confidence in nurses. Chesser-Smyth and Long (2013) posit that although there is little empirical evidence regarding self-confidence in nurses it is assumed to play a role in nurses' competence and is usually developed independently. "Self-confidence is the belief in one's abilities to accomplish a goal or task" (Potter & Perry 2001, as cited in Chesser-Smyth & Long, 2013, p. 146). New nurses require supportive environments with the major support coming from preceptors, managers, staff development, and team members. A lack of confidence can be detrimental to the new nurse and the preceptor plays a significant role in helping the nurse to become more confident. Preceptors must find a balance between acknowledging accomplishments and constructive criticism. Chesser-Smyth and Long (2013) found that new-nurse confidence eroded when they were subjected to poor preceptor attitudes, lack of communication, and felt undervalued. Almada et al. (2008) found a relationship between supportive work environments, length of orientation, and job satisfaction in new nurses. Ballard et al. (2012) posit that a weak orientation complicates what is already a challenging time for new nurses. They concluded that a disease-specific orientation leads to job satisfaction, clinical competence, and an improved knowledge base. Their study focused on a neurological unit; however, this type of orientation can be adapted for other types of units. Morris et al. (2009) evaluated a new model of critical care orientation that developed an individualized orientation based on assessment of critical thinking and competency development. They concluded that this model of orientation resulted in increased satisfaction and retention. They recommend that this model serve as a template throughout the hospital. These studies demonstrate the significance of the orientation program, especially in new nurses and nurses in specialty units.

Be sure to inform the powers that be if you require additional orientation. Most organizations realize the significance of providing new employees with a quality orientation and many will provide additional orientation and preceptorship for nurses who are making progress but would benefit from a few more weeks of support. Hospitals spend a lot of money on hiring and orienting new employees so it is in their best interest for you to be successful. Again, this is the time for you to be proactive and advocate for whatever you need to succeed.

GENERATIONAL ISSUES

Some studies have focused on generational issues and new-nurse preparedness. For example, Lampe et al. (2011) investigated orientation preferences of new-graduate nurses from Generation Y who were born after 1980 and have been described as "high maintenance" individuals who require constant and instantaneous feedback. The authors suggest that although all nurses may experience role stress they may require different types of support based on their generational influences. They further posit that preceptor selection may result in decreased role stress and improved satisfaction. They support a model in which a nurse preceptor from the same generational cohort and ethnicity be paired with the new orientee. This may present a challenge if the preceptor is fairly new to the organization, so they recommend using a more experienced preceptor for the second half of the orientation. Although this model has not been formally tested it does have merit. Generational differences have been the focus of turnover studies in nurses. For example, Takase (2006) found that nurses who were born between 1960 to 1974 viewed autonomy and recognition as important factors in their decision to change jobs, whereas nurses born after 1975 were more concerned with their ability to care for their patients. Nurses from different generations may have different perceptions regarding work environment (Sparks, 2012). Strategies to empower nurses should include generational differences. For example, Sparks (2012) found that baby boomers (1946–1964) value extrinsic rewards more than Generation X (1964–1980) does; however, both groups had similar psychological empowerment scores. Wieck (2005) found significant differences in baby boomers and Generation Xs in regard to support, autonomy, and job security with the latter valuing these more. Interestingly, new nurses, because of the various times of their lives into which they enter the profession, will often come from different generations, which may pose a challenge for hospital-based educators and leaders when developing an orientation program and selecting preceptors. Furthermore, you will be working with a group of diverse colleagues and caring for a diverse group of patients, both generationally and culturally, hence you must try to understand the various behaviors and norms of all the individuals you will be joining. For example, you may be technologically savvy because you grew up in an era of technology; however, individuals from past generations may not have that skill set. Therefore, keep an open mind and be patient when dealing with different people.

PRECEPTOR ISSUES

Preceptors play an important role in the development and acculturation of new nurses. Most hospitals use a preceptor-based orientation and assign an individual preceptor for every orientee. Many preceptors receive additional training and volunteer for this role. Sandau and Halm (2011) examined the effects of a preceptor class for preceptors and new orientees and found that the preceptors felt more prepared and confident in their roles; however, due to heavy patient workloads the new orientees were not satisfied with their experiences with their preceptors. Ideally, preceptors should be given a lighter assignment so they have adequate time to teach and coach you (Carlson et al., 2010). As you become more proficient the assignment may change, however, in the first few weeks, the preceptor should be able to spend a good portion of the day mentoring you. There are many wonderful preceptors who develop a special bond with their orientees. Unfortunately, not all preceptors are created equal and the role of the preceptor can be very challenging, especially when patient assignments are too heavy (Omansky, 2010). Most nurse preceptors desire to help new nurses, but at times may be overwhelmed. "Nurse preceptors experience role ambiguity, role conflict and role overload" (Omansky, 2010, p. 701). It is unfortunate and detrimental when organizations do not create a positive work environment and support their preceptors. Clearly, preceptors require education, experience, and support to excel at this challenging role. Although some preceptors receive small financial compensation, they do not do it for the financial gain; they do it because they are passionate about their profession and want to help new nurses assimilate into their roles. As a new nurse you want to be sensitive and understand that at times your preceptor may feel overwhelmed with trying to mentor you and still ensure all the needs of the patients are met, especially when the preceptor has a complex assignment.

Developing a positive relationship with your preceptor requires effort on both of your parts. As a new nurse you will need a lot of support and this can be very draining for the preceptor, especially when you first begin your orientation. Being an active participant in this relationship is very important. Try to avoid being an observer. Instead, take the initiative to assist your preceptor. Let your preceptor know your needs and be sure to show your appreciation for his or her support. You also need to understand that if the preceptor is feeling overwhelmed because of a challenging patient assignment or a patient suddenly becomes unstable he or she may not have time to explain things to you right at that moment. When this happens try to be as helpful as possible, take vital signs, assess your patients, and offer assistance to your preceptor. Be sure to use your self-efficacy and communication skills to promote a positive relationship. Your preceptor will be evaluating your progress and may have to offer constructive criticism, so try not to be too sensitive. The only way you are going to continue to develop and improve is to be open to suggestions given by your preceptor. Some preceptors do not know how to offer constructive criticism and their suggestions may come across as a reprimand or insult. If this happens, try to share your feelings with your preceptor as she or he may not realize how she or he is being perceived. According to Floyd (2003), many orientees perceive their preceptors to be "surrogate clinical instructors or spectators who only intervene when problems arise" (p. 26). It is helpful to discuss role expectations with your preceptor so you are both on the same page. Furthermore, the onus is on you to foster a collegial relationship with your preceptor and peers. As a new member to the group it takes time to develop a trusting relationship, hence you need to be patient and have realistic expectations of your preceptor and yourself. Eventually, you will find your comfort zone and build a trusting relationship with your colleagues. This happens at different times for different individuals, however, one day you will experience the "ah ha" moment when you feel like you are truly part of the team and have found your comfort zone. Many new graduates speak of this and although they do not always recognize when it happens suddenly they feel different, in a good way. Most new nurses will experience this epiphany during their first year.

Unfortunately, even if you do everything in your power to develop a positive relationship with your preceptor things just might not click between the two of you. If this happens you can try to talk to your preceptor; however, he or she may become defensive. Being an effective communicator is vital and you should review communication strategies that were discussed in Chapter 8. Be sure to think about what you want to say before you meet your preceptor and practice: videotaping your talking points and role playing can be helpful. You want to speak clearly and be assertive but not angry. Your tone should be even and nonaccusatory. Therefore, consider your verbal and nonverbal communication so that you are sending a clear message. Stay on topic and stick to the facts. Try not to be defensive. It can be very difficult to confront someone about his or her behavior so you need to choose your words wisely. Using the eight principles of "crucial conversations" (see Chapter 13) can be very helpful when dealing with sensitive issues. Sometimes it is best to have a mediator present, for example, your nurse manager or staff development coordinator, so that you can all discuss the situation in a professional manner. If the situation does not improve you may need to request a new preceptor. The orientation is vital to your success and you need a preceptor who will be supportive.

Top 10 Tips for New Nurses

1. Develop a strong knowledge base.
2. Commit to being a lifelong learner.
3. Develop mutual goals with your preceptor.
4. Develop a plan for the day.
5. Be proactive in your role.
6. Be an effective communicator.
7. Understand that it takes time to develop trusting relationships with colleagues.
8. Be sensitive to the needs of your preceptor.
9. Address issues in a professional manner.
10. Do not be afraid to ask for help.

Summary

This chapter focused on challenges you may face as a new nurse. Strategies for time management and organization were reviewed. A brief overview of reality shock, role stress, burnout, and job satisfaction was provided with strategies for prevention. Generational issues were briefly discussed as was the importance of being aware of differences among the generations. The role of the preceptor and strategies for a successful relationship were also discussed.

Discussion Questions

1. What strategies can you employ to improve time management?
2. What strategies can you employ to improve organizational skills?
3. What are the signs of burnout?
4. Identify antecedents of job satisfaction.
5. List and describe three ways to prevent burnout and role stress.
6. Discuss the positive and negative experiences of new graduates in regard to preceptors.

7. What strategies might you employ when dealing with a difficult preceptor?
8. Discuss findings from Takase et al. (2006) regarding generational issues and nurses.
9. Who might you reach out to if you are having issues with your preceptor or orientation program?
10. What are the time stealers identified by Cohen (2005)?

SUGGESTED LEARNING ACTIVITY

- Develop a time-management chart.
- Develop a plan for your day and evaluate whether you were able to follow it.
- Read three articles on role stress and/or burnout.
- Interview a nurse with at least 2 years of experience and another one with over 10 years of experience about their experiences as an orientee. Were they the same or different?
- Interview a preceptor about his or her role perceptions and ask whether he or she has any advice for orientees.

REFERENCES

Almada, P., Carafoli, K., Flattery, J. B., French, D. A., & McNamara, M. (2004). Improving the retention of newly graduated nurses. *Journal for Nurses in Staff Development, 20*(6), 268–273.

Ballard, J., Mead, C., Richardson, D., & Lotz, A. (2012). Impact of disease-specific orientation on new graduate nurse satisfaction and knowledge retention. *Journal of Neuroscience Nursing, 44*(3), 168–174. doi:10.1097/jnn.0b013e3182527465

Beecroft, P., Dorey. F., & Wenten, M. (2008). Turnover intention in new graduate nurses: A multivariate analysis. *Journal of Advanced Nursing, 62*(1), 41–52.

Benner, P. E. (1984). *From novice to expert: Excellence and power in clinical nursing practice.* Menlo Park, CA: Addison-Wesley.

Carlson, E., Pilhammar, E., & Wann-Hansson, C. (2010). Time to precept: Supportive and limiting conditions for precepting nurses. *Journal of Advanced Nursing, 66*(2), 432–441. doi:10.1111/j.1365-2648.2009.05174.x

Chesser-Smyth, P. A., & Long, T. (2013). Understanding the influences on self-confidence among first-year undergraduate nursing students in Ireland. *Journal of Advanced Nursing, 69*(1), 145–157. doi:10.1111/j.1365-2648.2012.06001.x

Clare, J., & Van Loon, A. (2003). Best practice principles for the transition from student to registered nurse. *Collegian, 10*(4), 25–31.

Cohen, S. (2005). Best of the basics. Reclaim lost time with better organization. *Nursing Management, 36*(10), 11.

Coomber, B., & Barriball, K. (2007). Impact of job satisfaction components on intent to leave and turnover for hospital-based nurses: A review of the research literature. *International Journal of Nursing Studies, 44,* 297–314.

Duchscher, J. (2009). Transition shock: The initial stage of role adaptation for newly graduated registered nurses. *Journal of Advanced Nursing, 65*(5), 1103–1113. doi:10.1111/j.1365-2648.2008.04898.x

Edwards, D. (2005). LTC employee turnover costs the nation billions every year. *Nursing Homes: Long Term Care Management, 54*(2), 16–24.

Floyd, J. (2003). How nurse preceptors influence new graduates. *Critical Care Nurse, 26.*

Kovner, C., Brewer, C., Fairchild, S., Poornima, S., Kim, H., & Djukic, M. (2007). Newly licensed RNs' characteristics, work attitudes, and intentions to work. *American Journal of Nursing, 107*(9), 58–70.

Lampe, K., Stratton, K., & Welsh, J. (2011). Evaluating orientation preferences of the Generation Y new graduate nurse. *Journal for Nurses in Staff Development, 27*(4), E6–9. doi:10.1097/NND.0b013e3182236646

Laschinger H. K., Finegan J., & Wilk, P. (2009). New graduate burnout: The impact of professional practice environment, workplace civility, and empowerment. *Nurse Economy, 27*(6), 377–383.

Lundgren, S., & Segesten, K. (2001). Nurses' use of time in a medical-surgical ward with all-RN staffing. *Journal of Nursing Management, 9*(1), 13–20. doi: 10.1046/j.1365-2834.2001.00192.x10.1111/j.1365-2834.2001.00192.x

Lynn, M., Morgan, J., & Moore, K. (2009). Development and testing of the satisfaction In nursing scale. *Nursing Research, 58*(3), 166–174.

Morris, L., Pfeifer, P., Catalano, R., Fortney, R., Nelson, G., Rabito, R., & Harap, R. (2009). Outcome evaluation of a new model of critical care orientation. *American Journal of Critical Care, 18*(3), 252–259. doi:10.4037/ajcc2009355

Omansky, G. (2010). Staff nurses' experiences as preceptors and mentors: An integrative review. *Journal of Nursing Management, 18*(6), 697–703. doi:10.1111/j.1365-2834.2010.01145.x

Sandau, K. E., & Halm, M. (2011). Effect of a preceptor education workshop, part 2: Qualitative results of a hospital-wide study. *Journal Of Continuing Education in Nursing, 42*(4), 172–181. doi:10.3928/00220124-20101101-02

Sparks, A. M. (2012). Psychological empowerment and job satisfaction between Baby Boomer and Generation X nurses. *Journal of Nursing Management, 20*(4), 451–460. doi:10.1111/j.1365-2834.2011.01282.x

Takase, M., Maude, P., & Manias, E. (2006). Role discrepancy: Is it a common problem among nurses? *Journal of Advanced Nursing, 54*(6), 751–759.

Thomack, B. (2012). Time management for today's workplace demands. *Workplace Health & Safety, 60*(5), 201–203. doi:10.3928/21650799-20120426-05

Thylefors, I. (2012). Does time matter? Exploring the relationship between interdependent teamwork and time allocation in Swedish interprofessional teams. *Journal of Interprofessional Care, 26*(4), 269–275. doi:10.3109/135618 20.2011.653609

Utriainen, K., & Kyngas, H. (2009). Hospital nurses' job satisfaction: A literature review. *Journal of Nursing Management, 17*(8), 1002–1010.

Watts, J., Robertson, N., Winter, R., & Leeson, D. (2013). Evaluation of organisational culture and nurse burnout. *Nursing Management—UK, 20*(6), 24–29.

Wieck, K. (2005). Generational approaches to current nursing issues: How younger and older nurses can coexist. *ISNA Bulletin, 31*(4), 27–30.

CHAPTER 15

Violence and Bullying in the Workplace

Knowing what's right doesn't mean much unless you do what's right.

— Theodore Roosevelt

I would rather be a little nobody, then to be an evil somebody.

— Abraham Lincoln

OBJECTIVES

After reading this chapter the reader will be able to:

- Identify types of bullying
- Understand critical social theory and oppressed groups
- Discuss The Joint Commission's standards on disruptive behaviors
- Understand the negative effects of bullying
- Discuss strategies for prevention of bullying/workplace violence

Bullying is a pervasive and damaging behavior that truly knows no boundaries. There are many different definitions of "bullying" and in health care organizations it is often referred to as workplace violence, lateral violence, horizontal violence, or disruptive behavior. No matter what it is called it does not change the fact that it is extremely negative and widespread and affects all professions, academic institutions, and people in general, especially vulnerable populations.

Bullying has been described as unwanted aggressive behavior that involves threats, rumors, physical and verbal abuse, and excluding individuals from the group with the behavior being repeated over and over (stopbullying.gov, 2014). "Examples of disruptive behaviors are throwing objects, banging down the telephone receiver, intentionally damaging equipment, and exposing patients or staff to contaminated fluids or equipment" (Lachman, 2014, p. 56). Victims may experience social isolation, depression, and despair and some resort to suicide. In recent years this issue has escalated, especially in school-age children and in health care organizations. In fact The Joint Commission (TJC, 2014) has implemented standards regarding disruptive behavior in the health care setting. Recognizing the seriousness of these issues, most organizations have adopted a "zero tolerance" policy. Many experts believe that people bully other people because they have low self-esteem. Critical social theory, which addresses oppressed groups, may demonstrate why "bullying" is so rampant among nurses. Historically, nurses—who are still predominately female—have been an oppressed group. Research demonstrates that oftentimes individuals who have been oppressed become the oppressors, hence a vicious cycle develops. Because bullying is so prevalent among nurses it is vital that you understand bullying and strategies you can employ to prevent it from happening. Furthermore, you want to be sure that you never become the "bully" because you were "bullied." As a new nurse you need to join your peers in ending this destructive cycle.

JOINT COMMISSION AND DISRUPTIVE BEHAVIORS

The issue of bullying escalated so much that The Joint Commission (2008) issued a sentinel event alert on disruptive behaviors and implemented leadership standards (TJC, 2009) to address these dangerous behaviors. Citing issues of poor patient satisfaction, potential adverse outcomes, and employee turnover this standard requires organizations to develop policies to prevent disruptive behaviors. Historically, disruptive behaviors have been ignored and underreported for fear of reprisal. Although the issue occurs in all disciplines and levels there is a higher incidence among individuals with power. Furthermore, some organizations ignore the behaviors of physicians who bring in high revenue (TJC, 2008). The Joint Commission (2008) identified the following behaviors as disruptive: threats, verbal outbursts, refusing to complete tasks, condescending attitudes, and refusal to return phone calls, or answer questions. The Joint Commission (2009) requires health care organizations to have a code of conduct and a process for managing disruptive behaviors. Furthermore, they encourage organizations to adopt a "zero tolerance" policy toward disruptive behaviors and to develop programs for patients and employees to address these negative behaviors. Despite these standards some employees are still afraid to report disruptive behavior for fear of losing their jobs, especially when it involves someone who is in a position of higher authority and power.

CRITICAL SOCIAL THEORY

Critical social theory may help one to understand the relationship of oppression and bullying/lateral/horizontal violence in the workplace. Throughout the years, nurses, health care workers, and patients have been oppressed by the paternalist medical model. In fact, Gordon (2005) recently highlighted that despite progress this pervasive issue still exists in our profession. Furthermore, as a historically oppressed group nurses need to be careful not become the oppressors in regard to patients and other staff members.

It is beneficial to understand critical social theory in regard to oppressed groups and vulnerable populations. In the 1920s a group of scholars from the Institute of Social Research, also known as the Frankfurt School, collaborated on the development of critical theory. The scholars came from various backgrounds but shared a similar vision in response to the technical knowledge being developed by logical positivistic science and oppression of the working class (How, 2003; Mohammed, 2006; Wilson-Thomas, 1994). "The critical social theory movement was aimed at rethinking the social philosophy of Marx. Marxism was grounded in an ideology of constraints based on class division and labor" (Wilson-Thomas, 1994, p. 573).

When Max Horkheimer assumed leadership of the school the philosophy shifted to culture instead of economics. Horkheimer wove subtle changes into Marx's assumptions. Horkheimer shifted away from the inductive approach and focused on a dialectical one. This approach linked insights of existentialism and economic reductionism (How, 2003). "Horkheimer insists that for a critical theory the world and subjectivity in all its forms have developed with the life processes of society" (Horkheimer 1982, p. 245, as cited in Bohman, 2005). According to Horkheimer critical theory must be explanatory, practical, and normative. The goal of critical social theory is to emancipate or free humans from the social and political circumstances that have enslaved them (Bohman, 2005). After World War II critical social theory lost its appeal as scholars moved to America.

In the late 1960s Jurgen Habermas was instrumental in rejuvenating the theory. Structure and social systems were now the focus. Jurgen Habermas is considered one of the most influential philosophers of all time. According to Habermas (1971), critical theory was used to generate knowledge. This is formed from free language that is not coerced. He discussed cognitive orientations, which were emancipatory, practical, and technical. The aim of critical social theory is to encourage self-reflection and unfreezing of one's assumptions that have been influenced by rules, habits, and traditions (Wilson-Thomas, 1995). "Habermas's theory is grounded in the Enlightenment tradition emphasizing reason, language, rational argument, a normative foundation for social critique, and a conception of history as moving in a dialectical manner towards emancipatory ideals" (Willette, 1998, as cited in Brown, 2000, p. 39). Emancipatory knowledge that promotes social change is the result of critically oriented science. Knowledge is created through the promotion of autonomy and responsibility that is free from oppressive coercion (Brown, 2000). Epistemological paradigms include: empirical–analytical, historical–hermeneutic, and critical social science. Habermas used these three approaches to acknowledge the value in generating intersubjective knowledge and predictive, technical knowledge. Moving beyond the constraints of each of these paradigms leads to emancipatory knowledge and social action. Emancipatory knowledge liberates individuals to make significant social change (Brown, 2000). Brown (2000) discussed the emergence of critical social theory, which was embraced by nurse scientists in the 1980s. There were several reasons for this movement, which related to the social and political factors that influenced health care of oppressed groups by a profession that was predominately female.

Fay (1987) defined critical social theory as a theory of self, society, and history. Critical social science assumes that humans are active creatures, or creatures who use their own self-interpretation to create themselves" (as cited in Dikinson, 1999, p. 146). First, the oppressive situation is uncovered, which enables victims to free themselves from the oppression (Dikinson, 1999).

Critical social theory was one of the theoretical approaches used to analyze empowerment in nursing. During their comprehensive literature search Kuokkanen and Leino-Kilpi (2000) identified categories of literature based on their theoretical orientation. One of the categories involved the use of critical social theory. Empowerment was viewed in regard to oppressed groups of women, racial minorities, and health care patients and the improvement of living conditions. Critical social theory often looks at this issue. An emancipatory starting point in nursing has been directed at nursing education. Some believe that empowered nurses are better able to empower their patients. Critical social theory in nursing is concerned with groups that are in a subordinated position, such as nurses and patients (Kuokkhanem & Leino-Kilpi, 2000). "Critical social theory is explicitly definable, stimulating and inspiring. It may prove useful in studies with ethical implications, for instance in research concerned with the priorities of nursing care" (Kuokkhanen & Leino-Kilpi, 2000, p. 239). Although the focus of this article was a concept analysis of empowerment the authors demonstrated the significant impact of critical social theory in regard to empowerment.

Mooney and Nolan (2005) wrote a critique of Freire's work on critical social theory in nursing education. Traditionally, nurses have been viewed as an oppressed group in relation to occupation, class, and gender. Furthermore, nursing education has perpetuated this oppression by the very nature of adhering to past traditions of teaching nursing. Freire's goal was to empower students and help them to be autonomous. According to Freire, praxis is the key to liberation. Critical praxis involves synchronized reflection and action. This enables an individual to identify and reflect on oppression, which in turn guides him or her toward liberation.

Oppression in nursing has been fostered by the use of the biomedical model and educators who continued to use traditional approaches to education. Oppression can lead to aggression and complaint that is directed within the group instead of at the oppressors. "Freire (1972) noted that the education process could act as a tool for conformity or an instrument for liberation and promoted an education based on liberation, whereby individuals are empowered through critical examination of their reality" (as cited in Mooney & Nolan, 2005, p. 241).

Another emphasis is on power relations of nurses and adolescent patients. Emancipation and equal partnerships should be embraced. This may prove difficult as nurses are usually in the dominant position. Empowering adolescents in their care can influence positive outcomes. The use of this theory helps nurses analyze issues and create social change (Mohammed, 2006).

Understanding critical social theory can help you to understand the possible underlying causes of bullying and the significance of empowering yourself and your patients. Although nurses are often at the receiving end of bullying, some are guilty of bullying or at the very least of incivility to other nurses and coworkers.

BULLYING, LATERAL AND HORIZONTAL VIOLENCE, AND INCIVILITY

Bullying, lateral and horizontal violence, and incivility are all terms that fall under the umbrella of disruptive behaviors. They are easily confused and often used interchangeably; however, they do have different connotations. "Bullying" is used broadly across all populations. Children and vulnerable populations are at greatest risk of experiencing bullying. As described above, bullying is repeated abusive behavior that occurs over a period of time and includes various types of threats, verbal and physical abuse, and excluding individuals from the group. In the health care setting bullying may appear as hostility, negative comments, and refusal to assist with tasks (Lachman, 2012).

"Tiberius and Flak (1999) characterized incivility as speech or action indicative of rudeness or lack of respect for those to whom such behavior is directed" (as cited in Robertson, 2012, p.21). Incivility is often written about in regard to students in an academic setting. Robertson (2012) described incivility and violence toward faculty in nursing and other higher education programs of study. Incivility has increased in recent years, causing some faculty to leave the profession. Robertson (2012) further posits that this issue is complex and exacerbated by stress and anxiety and the behaviors of students and faculty. Incivility in the health care setting may include rude behavior, condescending attitudes, screaming, name calling, and inappropriate jokes (Lachman, 2014).

"Lateral violence" and "horizontal violence" are terms used often to describe disruptive behaviors in the health care setting. Lateral violence pertains to the behavior of a person in power, such as a supervisor, administrator, manager, or physician, toward an employee such as a staff nurse, nursing assistant, or supervisor/subordinate (Growe, 2012). Horizontal violence pertains to the behavior of a person who works directly with the person and is at the same level, for example, nurse to nurse (Growe, 2012). This type of violence usually involves unkind or discourteous interactions, sarcasm, patronizing, and back biting (Lachman, 2012). Nurses who work in emergency rooms and psychiatric units are the most vulnerable to acts of violence committed by patients. However, physician violence against nurses also occurred, albeit on a smaller scale. Nurses report having objects thrown at them, being grabbed, being threatened, in addition to assaults of a sexual nature, such as fondling or light touching (Gordon, 2005). According to Becher and Visovsky (2012) negative relationships in the workplace may be related to burnout and poor patient outcomes. Horizontal violence has many negative effects and students and new nurses are frequently the targets. The negative effects of horizontal violence include depression, anxiety, turnover, powerlessness, anger, absenteeism, and negative patient outcomes (Becher & Visovsky, 2012). Growe (2012) posits that the American Nurses Association has "condemned workplace violence in any form against nurses" (p. 6); furthermore, "abusive behavior by a nurse is viewed as a violation of nursing ethics" (Growe, 2012, p. 6).

Some victims of bullying, especially vulnerable populations, may also turn to drugs and alcohol as a way to cope. As you can see, this is a very serious issue and you do not want to be on the receiving or the forwarding end of this type of behavior. Furthermore, although it may be difficult you certainly don't want to ignore this behavior because it may get worse. There are many strategies that can be employed to ameliorate this pervasive issue. For example, the organization must adopt a culture of civility and develop policies and education on positive behavior, teamwork and collaboration, and positive work environments. Knowing what constitutes bullying can help to empower nurses to stand up and advocate for themselves. Sometimes, a person who complains about bullying is called a whiner or complainer, or labeled as being overly sensitive. However, this is just another form of bullying. Treating someone in a negative way is never acceptable and must not be tolerated.

VIOLENCE IN THE WORKPLACE

Violence in the workplace is something that everyone must be prepared to experience. Although bullying, incivility, and horizontal and lateral violence may result in violent behavior, violence in the workplace may relate to a one-time incident by an employee, patient, or family member. This is a different type of disruptive behavior, which may arise from a confrontation and be more aggressive in nature. It often involves an aggressive act by a patient or family member to a caregiver. "Violence from patients should not be accepted as something that has to be tolerated by health care staff, and there needs to be strategies in place that send out clear messages to patients that such behaviour will not be accepted" (Bond, Paniagua, & Thompson, 2009, p. 99). Being alert to potential and sudden aggressive or violent behaviors is very important because many nurses and other health care professionals fall victim to this type of violent behavior. The Occupational Safety and Health Administration (OSHA, 2004) has developed guidelines for the prevention of violence in the workplace;

furthermore, employers are required to protect their employees from harm. According to OSHA (2004):

> BLS [Bureau of Labor Statistics] data shows that in 2000, 48 percent of all non-fatal injuries from occupational assaults and violent acts occurred in health care and social services. Most of these occurred in hospitals, nursing and personal care facilities, and residential care services. Nurses, aides, orderlies and attendants suffered the most non-fatal assaults resulting in injury. (p. 5)

As a new nurse you will want to become familiar with OSHA as this agency develops guidelines relating to many different types of employee protection. For example, in addition to protecting employees from harm they also have requirements for employers to create safe workplace environments for all their employees that also includes protection from hazardous materials and the provision of personal protective equipment.

The Crisis Prevention Institute (CPI; 2009) has developed a model for dealing with this type of behavior. The Crisis Prevention Institute (2009) defines a crisis as an event that occurs at a specific period in time and may result in a violent act. They recommend several strategies for preventing a crisis from developing or at least escalating. For example:

- Be a good listener
- Try not to be judgemental
- Maintain personal space
- Maintain a nonthreatening body stance
- Be aware of nonverbal and verbal communication
- Try to stay calm

According to their website the Crisis Prevention Institute offers specialized training in the safe management of disruptive and assaultive behavior. Following their guidelines may help to prevent a situation from escalating. Be sure to always follow your hospital's policies and contact your security department if you feel threatened in any way or by any person. Being prepared will help you to protect yourself from dangerous situations. Patients and families may become very stressed, anxious, and angry, which may be exacerbated if the situation is not handled correctly.

PREVENTING BULLYING

Bullying in any form is unacceptable and in the past few years bullying has escalated. For many years bullying was ignored or excused; however, this has been to our detriment as we have all watched in horror as the negative effect of bullying has reared its ugly head with escalating violence that has resulted in murders, suicides, and severe injuries. Today many organizations are addressing bullying and disruptive behaviors; however, we still have a long way to go.

There are many strategies that can be employed to address this issue. Having a "zero tolerance" policy sends a strong message to potential and actual abusers. However, in order for this to be effective it must be enforced and victims must be empowered to report issues of abuse. Empowerment is a key strategy for dealing with bullying. Having a support system is also crucial and can make a big difference in how a situation is addressed. Yang et al. (2013) described the applicability of Kanter's Theory of Structural Power in Organizations and empowerment of nurses. Power is the ability to get things done, with formal power relating to role and informal power arising from having supportive relationships.

Take, for example, Dorothy in the Wizard of Oz. The Wizard of Oz is a fictional story about Dorothy, a young girl whose house is caught up in a tornado and lands on top of the Wicked Witch in the Land of Oz. Throughout the story Dorothy tries to find a way back home to her family. This story had victims and bullies. The victims, at least in the beginning, were Dorothy, the Scarecrow, the Tin Man, and the Cowardly Lion. The Cowardly Lion is a perfect example of a bully who has low self-esteem, and what happens when someone stands up to this type of person. At first the Cowardly Lion is mean and aggressive; however, when Dorothy confronts him he cries and becomes meek. Eventually, the Cowardly Lion, the Scarecrow, and the Tin Man join together to help each other find the Wizard of Oz, who they hope will be able to help them. Along the way they meet the real bully, the other Wicked Witch, who vows revenge on Dorothy because she killed her sister. Naturally, everyone is frightened of the Wicked Witch; however there is also a good witch called Glinda who is a supporter and advocate, and encourages the group to stand up to the Wicked Witch. Eventually, the group bands together and defeats the Wicked Witch. At the end of the story Dorothy realizes that she possesses the power to find her way back home. This story is a perfect depiction of what one can do when faced with adversity. You have to identify the issues, find supportive individuals, and face your fears.

Knowing the organization's policies and procedures is very important as then you will know exactly what to do if faced with disruptive behavior. Remember that organizations are required to address disruptive behavior in accordance with The Joint Commission and OSHA. Furthermore, nurses are expected to follow their Code of Conduct, which explicitly addresses the avoidance of creating a negative work environment. Gordon (2005) discussed the significance of whistle-blower protection and the role of unions in protecting the rights of employees. Another example provided by Gordon (2005) is a program implemented by the Swiss Nurses Association and the Federation des Infirmiers et Inirmieres de Quebec (FIIQ). As part of this program nurses were provided with pocket-sized cards imprinted with advice on dealing with hostile environments. For example, one card contains the following advice (Gordon, 2005, p. 427):

> I am empowering myself to eliminate violence in the workplace.
>
> 1. I take a deep breath; I trust myself.
> 2. I tell the person: "I do not accept this behavior" and give them the red card.
> 3. Report the incident to the hotline (a call-in number the union has established).
> 4. Inform your union representative.

This is just one example, but it supports the premise that nurses must be empowered to address the negative behavior of colleagues, physicians, and supervisors. Laschinger and Wong (2006) addressed the issue of workplace empowerment as a way to improve work environment and decrease the nursing shortage. The study looked at staff nurse perceptions about empowerment and nursing burnout. "Stressful working conditions in nursing are a major cause of burnout among nurses. Burnout is characterized by exhaustion, cynicism, and low professional efficacy" (Laschinger & Wong, 2006, p. 358). Educational workshops can be offered by organizations to help nurses and other staff members improve their self-efficacy and empowerment skills. "The theory of self-efficacy states that perceived self-efficacy, defined as an individual's judgment of his or her capabilities to organize and execute courses of action, is a determinant of performance" (Peterson & Bredow, 2004, p. 104). Enhancing self-efficacy in nursing may influence the nurse to improve professional practice (Manojlovich, 2005). Resiliency and self-advocacy are also important factors in developing and enhancing coping skills, empowerment, and self-efficacy. Similar to a knight donning his coat of armor, these skills can offer protection against the negative effects of bullying and help you to find the courage to address the many behaviors associated with bullies.

You should always follow your chain of command and never be put off by a particular individual because everyone has a supervisor who oversees his or her work. If you exhaust the chain of command you do have the right to contact The Joint Commission, OSHA, your union representative, and whatever organizations are available in your location. Furthermore, if you feel you have been wrongly accused or terminated because you reported disruptive behavior you should seek legal counsel. You may advocate for yourself or others and be sure to understand whistle-blower laws and the protection they offer when reporting adverse issues in your organization. Whistle-blower laws relate to issues that are either morally, ethically, and, more importantly, legally wrong. In the United States, OSHA enforces the whistle-blower statutes to protect employees from retaliation.

The Occupational Safety and Health (OSH) Act prohibits employers from discriminating against their employees for exercising their rights under the OSH Act. These rights include filing an OSHA complaint, participating in an inspection or talking to an inspector, seeking access to employer exposure and injury records, and raising a safety or health complaint with the employer. If workers have been retaliated or discriminated against for exercising their rights, they must file a complaint with OSHA within 30 days of the alleged adverse action (OSHA, 2014).

It is important to understand and be knowledgeable about the laws that govern and protect employees. Because different countries have different guidelines you should be sure to research all the organizations and laws that have been implemented to protect you from bullying and other negative issues that may jeopardize your employment and license to practice. Remember the following quote so that you always advocate for yourself and others:

> If you are neutral in situations of injustice, you have chosen the side of the oppressor. If an elephant has its foot on the tail of a mouse, and you say that you are neutral, the mouse will not appreciate your neutrality.
>
> — *Desmond Tutu*

Top 10 Ways to Address Bullying

1. Be knowledgeable about the different types of bullying and workplace violence.
2. Review your organization's policies on these disruptive behaviors.

3. Be well versed in the guidelines and standards of regulatory agencies.
4. Develop your self-efficacy and empowerment skills.
5. Use the eight principles of "crucial conversations" when dealing with bullies.
6. Report all incidences of bullying through proper channels.
7. Understand how critical social theory relates to bullying.
8. Collaborate with your colleagues to create a positive work environment.
9. Embrace a "zero tolerance" approach to bullying.
10. Continually monitor your behavior so you don't become a bully.

SUMMARY

This chapter focused on the pervasive and negative impact of bullying and violence in the workplace. A discussion of the types of bullying and workplace violence that may occur was included. Critical social theory as a possible explanation of workplace violence, especially horizontal violence in nurses, was reviewed. An overview of strategies on ways to deal with this type of behavior was provided, in addition to available supports such as OSHA, The Joint Commission, employee unions, and hospital administrators.

DISCUSSION QUESTIONS

1. What is bullying?
2. Discuss the negative effects of bullying.
3. What is incivility?
4. Compare and contrast horizontal and lateral violence?
5. What are the strategies recommended by the Crisis Prevention Institute when dealing with potentially aggressive individuals?
6. Discuss strategies you can employ to address disruptive behaviors.

7. What is the position of The Joint Commission and OSHA in regards to bullying?
8. What is self-efficacy?
9. What are the four pieces of advice nurses are given to deal with hostile environments?
10. What other strategies might you employ to protect yourself from bullies?

Suggested Learning Activities

- Role play scenarios relating to workplace violence.
- Complete an online checklist of your self-efficacy skills.
- Research The Joint Commission and OSHA or other agencies in your country or province regarding bullying and whistle-blowing.
- Interview at least three nurses about whether they have been bullied. Be sure to ask them how they handled the situation and what advice they would offer to a victim of bullying and/or violence in the workplace.

REFERENCES

Becher, J., & Visovsky, C. (2012). Horizontal violence in nursing. *MEDSURG Nursing, 21*(4), 210–214.

Bohman, J., 1991. New Philosophy of Social Science: Problems of Indeterminacy, Cambridge: MIT Press

Bohman, J. (2005). Critical theory. In E. N. Zalta (Ed.), *The Stanford encyclopedia of philosophy*. Stanford, CA: Stanford University. Retrieved from http://plato.stanford.edu/archives/spr2005/entries/critical-theory

Bond, P., Paniagua, H., & Thompson, A. (2009). Zero tolerance of violent patients: policy in action. *Practice Nursing, 20*(2), 97–99.

Browne, A. (2000). The potential contributions of critical theory to nursing science. *Canadian Journal of Nursing Research, 32*(2), 35–55.

Crisis Prevention Institute. (2009). *CPI capsule. Ten tips for preventing a crisis.* Retrieved from https://www.crisisprevention.com

Dikinson, J. (1999). A critical social theory approach to nursing care of adolescents with diabetes. *Issues in Comprehensive Pediatric Nursing, 22*, 143–152.

Fay, B. (1987). *Critical social science: Liberation and its limits.* Ithaca, NY: Cornell University Press.

Gordon, S. (2005). *Nursing against the odds: How health care cost cutting, media stereotypes, and medical hubris undermine nurses and patient care.* New York: Cornell University Press.

Growe, S. (2013). Bullying/lateral violence/horizontal violence/disruptive behavior in the workplace. *Nevada Reformation, 22*(1), 6.

Habermas, J. (1971). *Knowledge and Human Interests.* Boston: Beacon Press.

How, A. (2003). *Critical theory.* New York, NY: Palgrave.

The Joint Commission. (2008). *Behaviors that undermine a culture of safety. Sentinel event alert, issue 40.* Retrieved from http://www.jointcommission .org/assets/1/18/SEA_40.pd

The Joint Commission. (2009). *Disruptive behaviors.* Retrieved at https://www .jointcommision.org

Kuokkanen, L., & Leino-Kilpi, H. (2000). Power and empowerment in nursing: Three theoretical approaches. *Journal of Advanced Nursing, 31*(1), 235–241.

Lachman, V. D. (2014). Ethical issues in the disruptive behaviors of incivility, bullying, and horizontal/lateral violence. *MEDSURG Nursing, 23*(1), 56–60.

Laschinger, H. K., & Wong, C. A. (2006). The impact of staff nurse empowerment on person–job fit and work engagement/burnout. *Nurse Administration Quarterly, 30*(4), 358–367.

Manojolovich, M. (2005). Promoting nurses' self-efficacy: A leadership strategy to improve practice. *Journal of Nursing Administration, 35*(5), 271.

Mohammed, S. (2006). Re-examining health disparities: Critical social theory in pediatric nursing. *Journal for Specialists in Pediatrics, 11*(1), 68–71.

Mooney, M., & Nolan, L. (2006). A critique of Freire's perspective on critical social theory in nursing education. *Nurse Education Today, 26,* 240–244.

Occupational Safety and Health Administration. (2004). *Guidelines for preventing workplace violence for health care & social service workers.* Retrieved from https://www.osha.gov

Occupational Safety and Health Administration. (2014). *The whistle blower protection programs.* Retrieved from https://www.whistleblowers.gov/

Peterson, S., & Bredow, T. (2004). *Middle range theories application to nursing research.* Philadelphia, PA: Lippincott, Williams & Wilkins.

Robertson, J. E. (2012). Can't we all just get along? A primer on student incivility in nursing education. *Nursing Education Perspectives, 33*(1), 21–26. doi:10.5480/1536-5026-33.1.21

Stopbullying.gov. (2014). *What is bullying?* Retrieved from https://www.stop-bullying.gov

Tiberius, R. G., & Flak, E. (1999). Incivility in dyadic teaching and learning. *New Directions for Teaching and Learning, 77,* 3–12. doi: 10.1002/tl.7701

Willette, C. (1998). Practical discourse as policy making: An application of Habermas' discourse ethics within a community mental health setting. *Canadian Journal of Community Mental Health, 17*(2), 27–38.

Wilson-Thomas, L. (1995). Applying critical social theory in nursing education to bridge the gap between theory, research and practice. *Journal of Advanced Nursing, 21,* 568–575.

Yang, J., Liu, Y., Huang, C., & Zhu, L. (2013). Impact of empowerment on professional practice environments and organizational commitment among nurses: A structural equation approach. *International Journal of Nursing Practice, 18,* 44–55. doi:10.1111/ijn.12016

CHAPTER 16

Journaling

Without deep reflection one knows from daily life that one exists for other people.

—Albert Einstein

OBJECTIVES

After reading this chapter the reader will be able to:

- Identify the relationship of journaling and successful transitions
- Know how to journal
- Discuss types of journals and their key components
- Use journaling as a means of reflection
- Understand the benefits of journaling

Nursing is an extremely rewarding and at times a rather stressful profession. In previous chapters the benefits of journaling were briefly mentioned. The literature contains a plethora of evidence to support the use of journaling for self-reflection and as a means of catharsis for nursing students and nurses (Epp, 2008).

> Journaling is a process by which a person engages in self-reflection through written accounts of positive and negative personal experiences. Through the process of critical self-reflection a person may reflect on the meaning of what has been learned and expand their worldview. (Hunt, 2013, p. 288)

It is important to note that there is no right or wrong way to journal, except if it is part of an assignment for which your teacher has provided guidelines. A journal is a private and personal item and your thoughts are sacred. You should only share you journal if you feel comfortable doing so. If a journal is part of a formal assignment you may be asked to share themes of your writings, but not the actual journal. This way you can decide what you feel comfortable sharing. Because journaling has so many benefits it is strongly recommended that you keep a journal during your student days and when you enter the world of professional nursing. The guidelines and information contained in this chapter are offered to guide you in the process; however, once you embrace the process you will find ways to develop your own unique way of journaling.

KEEPING A JOURNAL

Journaling is the act of writing or recording one's innermost thoughts and feelings on a particular experience or subject. Some individuals keep a journal because they like to write or they enjoy looking back at their experiences. Others keep a journal for professional or academic reasons. Some may use it for self-development or self-reflection. The wonderful thing about journaling, especially if it is not assigned, is that you decide the how, why, when, and where of this experience. For example, you may choose to write, type, or record your feelings. You might do this every day, once per week, a few times per month, or sporadically. It is totally up to you. This in itself is very liberating and empowering. Your reasons for keeping a journal may be for self-reflection, self-development, or just because this is something you enjoy. You might write a journal at home, or on the train, or during your break time at work. Perhaps you only write when you are very upset or have a really unique experience. Charles (2010) indicates that the literature is mixed when supporting the benefits of journaling; however, it is widely used. She further recommends that journaling should be done in free form with no guidelines or restrictions. Some individuals purchase a special book or notebook to record their feelings and experiences in, whereas others write down thoughts on index cards or pieces of scrap paper. Using your computer is also an option as typing may be preferred to written notes. A tape recorder can be a good option, and there are programs that turn voice to text, so if you want to have a written document you can. A journal is a very personal and private account and you should use whatever tools you prefer.

JOURNALING AND SELF-REFLECTION

Reflective journaling is a specific type of journaling in which one reflects on the situation, the experience, and his or her thoughts and feelings. One may also consider whether he or she would act the same way in a similar situation. Journaling helps one to reflect and understand the meaning of events (Kerka, 2002). Schuessler et al. (2012) examined the relationship of journaling, self-reflection, and the development of cultural humility in nursing students. They found that with each semester the students became more sensitive to cultural differences.

The use of reflective journaling (Blake, 2005) and narrative pedagogy (Brown, Kirkpatrick, Mangum, & Avery, 2008), has been embraced by many nurse educators in undergraduate and graduate programs in an attempt to enhance critical thinking, self-awareness, and self-development (Grendell, 2011, as cited in Hunt, 2013, p. 287).

Self-reflection is something many of us engage in as a subconscious act. However, a journal is a more formal and deliberate process for pursuing self-reflection and is useful for students and nurses. There are so many experiences—some positive and some negative—and you should reflect on both of these. For example, if you have a perfect day when everything went well and you are proud of your accomplishments, you want to reflect on this experience so you can figure out what factors were related to it. The next time you are faced with a similar situation you can take the same approach. On the other hand, if you have a negative or particularly stressful day you can reflect on what you might have done differently to handle this type of situation.

Some days you may feel disappointed and filled with self-doubt because you did not meet your own expectations. Reflection can help you to analyze the events of the day—oftentimes things may not seem as bad after you have had time to reflect and evaluate. For example, perhaps your expectations were unrealistic, or you didn't have the tools you needed to accomplish your tasks. Furthermore, emotions are usually more stable several hours after an event has occurred. Journaling can help students deal with some of the fears they face when caring for challenging patients, such as in a psychiatric unit (Waldo & Hermans, 2009). "A common theme in much of the journaling literature relates to an enhanced understanding of the self through reflection" (Lepp et al., 2005, p. 53).

Participating in the act of journaling can help you to see things in a new light and develop new perspectives and a higher order of reflection and self-awareness. In support of this, Lepp et al. (2005) concluded, "This greater self-awareness, as a deeper personal knowing, results in professional socialization and the development of mature human skills, such as empathy, understanding, as well as verbal and nonverbal communication" (p. 57).

As a nurse you will deal with the human experience and the emotions of your patients and yourself. On any given day you might encounter a patient and/or family who is joyful and happy, angry and depressed, sorrowful or despondent, anxious and stressed, frustrated or exuberant, grateful or unappreciative, or in a stage of acceptance or denial. As a human being who is sharing this experience you may have similar experiences and may feel the same way at times. Therefore, it is imperative you have an outlet and a way to deal with these emotions. Journaling can be very helpful in processing the myriad emotions you will have on a daily basis. You can also encourage your patients and families to journal to help them deal with the negative and positive experiences related to their health and wellness. Lepp et al. (2005) found that when students engaged in journaling they were able to engage in self-reflection, which increased their self-awareness. Journaling may also help nurses to develop their ability to presence themselves with their patients. Presencing has been discussed frequently in the literature and Benner (1984) is one of the well-known experts who identified presencing as an important ability in nurses. Benner (1989) states, "This ability to presence oneself, to be with a patient in a way that acknowledges shared humanity, is the base of nursing as a caring practice. . . . To presence oneself with another means understanding and being with someone" (as cited in Thompson, 2005, p. 465).

Wright (2001) described the "clear-eyed" nurse and the "cloudy-eyed" nurse, with the latter type giving the patient his or her full attention, which helps them to heal.

Although Benner (1984) and Wright (2001) did not discuss the relationship of journaling and presencing, and no studies were located to support this premise, this author believes that because presencing requires one to understand and be in the moment with someone it seems plausible that journaling would enhance this skill. There truly is a difference between caring for someone and caring with presencing; patients certainly realize when you are just going through the motions of care versus truly sharing their experiences, both positive and negative.

BENEFITS OF JOURNALING FOR SELF-DEVELOPMENT

Journaling as a tool for self-development has been widely embraced by many disciplines, including nursing (Charles, 2010; Fritson, Forrest, & Bowl, 2011). This type of journaling may be required and assigned by a faculty member, although one can still do this type of journaling on her or his own. If this is part of an assignment, your faculty member will provide clear guidelines as to how to complete the journal. You may be required to share some parts or your entire journal for this type of assignment. Furthermore, your teacher will be providing feedback to you throughout the process. Journaling commonly results in enhanced self-understanding, professional development, and self-renewal (Lepp et al., 2005, p. 53). Clearly, the many benefits of journaling cannot be ignored. In a more recent study Kuo et al. (2011) found that "journaling in nursing students was related to self-confidence, self-development, caring behaviors, ability to reflect, and improvement in writing abilities" (p. 141).

Journaling may be used for spiritual growth, meditation, and reflection on one's spiritual beliefs. It may provide a safe and private way for an individual to question his or her religion or the existence of a higher power in light of all the suffering a nurse sees in patients and experiences in his or her own life. It may also be used as a catharsis to address negative feelings and experiences. For example, you might have to care for a patient who committed a heinous crime and it will be challenging to be empathetic and caring in this situation. Writing and reflecting on what you write in your journal may help you come to terms with your feelings. Carley (2012) posits that journaling may reduce grief and depression and enhance relationships with patients, families, and coworkers. In her study on journaling and NICU (neonatal intensive care) families, she found a relationship between family journaling and stress reduction. Although many studies focus on the benefits to the nurse or other health care professional, this study demonstrates the potential benefits of journaling in patients and/or families.

You might use journaling when dealing with a bully or difficult coworker as the act of writing and reflection may help you to figure out the best way to deal with this type of situation (Waldo, 2005). It may also help you to let go of your feelings (Evers, 2004). Writing down your feelings is related to decreased anger (Carley, 2012), which may be helpful when processing the negative effects of bullying and when confronting a bully.

The art of keeping a journal may help to improve writing skills and creativity, which will help you to further develop your ability to write in a more scholarly manner. In fact many writers use journals to help them develop ideas and also deal with writer's block. Nurses have so many stories to share and the act of keeping a journal will certainly help you in your future publications, which may relate to personal or scholarly works, in addition to the academic writing you will be required to complete as you continue your education.

Blake (2005) identified several areas identifying the educational benefits of journaling, which include discovering meaning in an experience, making connections between theory and practice, instilling values such as altruism, understanding perspectives of patients, reflecting on the nursing role, improving writing and critical-thinking skills, developing affective skills such as empathy, and the ability to care for oneself in response to human suffering (as cited in Hunt, 2013, p. 268).

Narrative pedagogy is related to journaling and is used in some nursing programs. It requires in-depth analysis of a situation and may enhance problem solving and critical thinking in students (Grendell, 2000). Narrative pedagogy involves a formal process and your faculty may develop teaching and learning strategies based on it. It is similar to the type of journaling that is used for self-reflection and your faculty member will provide you with specific guidelines and a grading rubric to help you learn how to engage in this type of learning.

JOURNALING FOR TRANSITION

Engaging in journaling as you transition into professional practice can be very beneficial. As previously discussed, the transition period can be very challenging and stressful and journaling can provide you with a means to reflect on these challenges. For example, Washington (2012) found that journaling was related to decreased anxiety in graduate nurses. Sewell (2008) supports the use of journals for nursing students and new-graduate nurses as they transition into their professional practice roles. Lepp et al. (2005) found that journaling helped new nurses transition and enhanced their socialization into the profession. Journaling provides an outlet for the myriad feelings you will experience as a nurse, especially during your transition.

The death of a patient often results in mixed feelings. For example, the unexpected death of a patient, especially a child or infant, is very sad and although it never gets easy the first one is the most difficult. On the other hand, based on your culture and spirituality, you may not view death in a negative way and find it hard to understand why many individuals experience an emotional and physical breakdown when their loved ones pass away. Analyzing your feelings through the words in your journal may help you to deal with your emotions and understand the feelings of your patients and/or family members. Lasater and Nielson (2009) found that reflective journaling with specific guidelines was correlated with positive student-learning outcomes. "We discovered valuable student learning, improved evaluation of clinical thinking, and enhanced communication about clinical judgment development were the outcomes when a reflective guide and developmental rubric, rooted in an evidence-based conceptual framework, were used" (Lasater & Nielson, 2009, p. 44). Considering the benefits of these practices new nurses should also be expected to participate in reflective journaling, with guides being provided by hospital-based educators. Blake (2005) described the many benefits of journaling, narrative pedagogy, and self-reflection. These benefits include discovering the meaning of a particular experience and helping one to understand what it means and how it informs or undergirds his or her life and nursing care. Another benefit is the making of connections between theoretical concepts and clinical experiences.

The relationship of reflection and the professional role can lead to greater insight and empowerment. Journaling may also lead to improvement of writing skills and the development of critical thinking, effective skills, and the ability to care for self and others.

There are many personal and professional benefits related to journaling. Journaling offers personal growth and development and the development of a worldview. It may also have a positive effect on patients who benefit from practitioners who are better prepared to provide holistic, therapeutic, and competent nursing care. Initially, it may require practice and perseverance to write in your journal, however, with time it will become a part of your normal routine. Journaling will serve you well as a student and a nurse.

Another benefit that has not been discussed is the ability to look back in time, read about your experiences, relate it to your current role and reflect on how much you have learned and developed. You may find some entries humorous, inspiring, frustrating, or sad. You may wonder why you felt so upset about an incident because now that some time has passed the issue seems trivial. You may be very proud of yourself as you realize how many peoples' lives you have touched along the way. Reading your old journal entries may serve as a reminder to get back on track with your plans for your academic and professional growth. Perhaps, when you first became a nurse you made a plan to return to school within 2 years. However, now looking back at your journal entries, 4 years have passed and you still have not returned to school, or obtained a particular certification. On the other hand, you may have accomplished all of your personal and professional goals and although you are proud of yourself you realize it is time to develop some new goals. In summary, journaling has many benefits and is particularly useful for students and new nurses during the transition period.

KEY COMPONENTS OF A JOURNAL

A journal may be completed as a formal assignment as a student, but for the most part journals are unique to the individual. A journal is a personal narrative and may include written words, pictures, drawings, and electronic writings (Carley, 2012). It is a private and personal experience and it should be viewed as something sacred. Some people like to purchase a plain notebook and decorate it. The key is to use something that has special meaning to you and that others know they should not read.

Some people like to develop a routine for their journaling. Routine is a concept that pertains to behavioral patterns that are used to organize and coordinate activities. Maintaining a personal routine may assist people through life-changing events (Zisberg et al., 2007). Therefore, you may want to journal at a particular time or day and set aside a special time for you to write in your journal. Or you may decide to journal only on the days you find stressful or experience something new. Unless this is part of a formal assignment you can do whatever you want when it comes to journaling; however, if you want to realize some of the benefits that were discussed in this chapter you will need to develop a more formalized routine for your journaling.

You will also need to decide how and when you will reflect on your journal. For example, you may decide to reflect on your journal once a week or once a month. It will depend on how often you journal and what you are hoping to accomplish. Unless this is a formal assignment the length of the entries is totally up to you. It can be a few sentences to a couple of pages. It really depends on the experiences and your thoughts at the time. For many individuals the words just flow after they jot down the first sentence. One key to journaling is to do it in a place where you will not be disturbed or anxious that someone will try to look over your shoulder and read what you have written because that will block your thoughts. Try not to become frustrated if you can only write a few words as this process should help you to relax—not cause you to have more stress. You may find the 10 tips included at the end of this chapter and the sample assignment suggested in the Appendix helpful as you write and reflect on your journal entries. Doing a relaxation exercise with a brief meditation or some deep cleansing breaths may help you to clear you mind and center yourself prior to writing in your journal. One tip listed below is to include your senses—what did you see, hear, feel, smell, or taste? For example, did you see human suffering or joy? Did you see someone do something that really affected you? This could be something positive or negative.

For example, did you observe a practitioner not following safety protocols? You may have been very upset but not sure how to confront the person. Or did you hear your patient crying, laughing, or yelling? On a more personal note, did you hear a tone in your voice that communicated annoyance or anger directed toward your patients or colleagues? Did you feel joy, sadness, anger, frustration, or perhaps you felt that in your patients and families? Did you offer a healing/caring touch to someone in need? Or perhaps someone offered you that healing touch?

Did you smell something so awful that you never hope to smell it again? Or encounter something so beautiful, like a newborn baby, that brought you joy and good feelings? Did you taste your own tears as you grieved for a patient or cried due to a personal experience? You may use your senses while writing and then later while reflecting on your experiences. This can help you to consider what you might do the same or differently next time you encounter a similar situation.

To conclude, these are guidelines you might want to consider when partaking in the art of journaling. Indeed, there is no right or wrong way to journal and this is a very personal and unique experience. If you are journaling for an assignment you will need to follow the guidelines developed by your instructor, however, this is still a personal and unique experience and you have the final say in what and how much you will share.

Top 10 Tips for Journaling

1. Date your entries.
2. Find a quiet place to write in your journal.
3. Meditate and center yourself before you write.
4. Consider purchasing a special book or journal to write in.
5. Write about your experiences both positive and negative (e.g., the transition, working on the unit, etc.).
6. Use your senses—what was the experience like?
7. Reflect on these experiences.
8. Consider what you would have done differently.
9. Write about your patient encounters, the first time you did something, your relationships with preceptor, colleagues, and peers.
10. Reflect on your journal and identify its major themes.

SUMMARY

This chapter focused on the art and benefits of journaling. An overview of journaling and ways to journal were provided. The many benefits of journaling were discussed, which include self-development, stress reduction, knowledge development, writing skills, and socialization into the profession. The benefits of journaling during transition were briefly discussed in addition to the use of narrative pedagogy. Self-reflection and self-development were described in relation to journaling.

DISCUSSION QUESTIONS

1. What is the art of journaling?
2. Why is it helpful to journal?
3. How does journaling relate to self-development?
4. What is the relationship of journaling and self-reflection?
5. List and discuss three benefits of journaling.
6. What are some ways you may journal?
7. What should you include in your journal?
8. What is narrative pedagogy?
9. Discuss the benefits of presencing.
10. How might journaling help you address bullying?

SUGGESTED LEARNING ACTIVITIES

- Keep a journal for at least 3 months as a student and as a nurse and reflect on the benefits.
- Reflect on your journal entries using the narrative pedagogy assignment in the Appendix.
- Interview two nurses who journal.
- Conduct a literature search on the benefits of journaling and write an essay.
- Begin a journal club at your school or organization.

APPENDIX

Sample Assignment — Pediatric Experience

Narrative Pedagogy (20%)
Describe:

- The clinical situation (patient, staff, environment)
- Your situation with the patient and family
- Your concerns at the time
- QSEN (Quality and Safety Education for Nurses) competencies in relation to your situation
- Patient safety

Reflect on:

- Your thoughts as the situation was unfolding
- Your feelings during and after the situation
- What was the most challenging, most rewarding?
- Important conversations you had with the patient, family, staff, and others
- What you would have done differently?
- Other important factors

Discuss:

- Share this reflection with group*
- Current analysis of situation
- Lessons learned

REFERENCES

Benner, P. (1984). *From novice to expert: Excellence and power in clinical nursing practice.* Menlo Park, CA: Addison-Wesley.

Benner, P., & Wrubel, J. (1989). *The primacy of caring: Stress and coping in health and illness.* Menlo Park, CA: Addison-Wesley.

Blake, T. (2005). Journaling: An active learning technique. *International Journal of Nursing Education Scholarship, 2*(1) 1–13.

Brown S. T., Kirkpatrick M. K., Mangum D., & Avery J. A review of narrative pedagogy strategies to transform traditional nursing education. *Journal of Nursing Education, 47*(7), 283–286.

Carley, A. (2012). Can journaling provide support for NICU families? *Journal for Specialists in Pediatric Nursing, 17*(3), 254–257. doi:10.1111/j.1744-6155.2012.00336.x

---

* Only share what you are comfortable sharing with the group.

Charles, J. (2010). Journaling: creating space for "i." *Creative Nursing, 16*(4), 180–184. doi:10.1891/1078-4535.16.4.180

Epp, S. (2008). The value of reflective journaling in undergraduate nursing education: A literature review. *International Journal of Nursing Studies, 45*(9), 1379–1388. doi:10.1016/j.ijnurstu.2008.01.006

Evers, F. T. (2008). Journaling: A path to our innermost self. *Interbeing, 2*(2), 53–56.

Fritson, K. K., Forrest, K. D., & Bohl, M. L. (2011). *Using reflective journaling in the college course.* Dubuque, IA: APA Division 2, Society for the Teaching of Psychology.

Grendell, R. N. (2011). Narrative pedagogy, technology, and curriculum transformation in nursing education. *Journal of Leadership Studies, 4*(4), 65–67. doi:10.1002/jls.20197

Hunt, D. (2013). *The New nurse educator: Mastering academe.* New York: Springer Publishing.

Lasater, K., & Nielsen, A. (2009). Reflective journaling for clinical judgment development and evaluation. *Journal of Nursing Education, 48*(1), 40–44. doi:10.3928/01484834-20090101-06

Lepp, M., Zorn, C., Duffy, P., & Dickson, R. (2005). Swedish and American nursing students use journaling for reflection: An international student-centered learning experience. *International Journal for Human Caring, 9*(4), 52–58.

Kerka, S. (2002). Journal writing as an adult learning tool. Retrieved from https://www.calpro-online.org/eric/docs/pab00031.pdf

Kuo, C., Turton, M., Cheng, S., & Lee-Hsieh. (2011). Using clinical caring journaling: Nursing student and instructor experiences. *Journal of Nursing Research, 19*(2), 141–149.

Schuessler, J. B., Wilder, B., & Byrd, L. W. (2012). Reflective journaling and development of cultural humility in students. *Nursing Education Perspectives, 33*(2), 96–99. doi:10.5480/1536-5026-33.2.96

Sewell, E. (2008). Journaling as a mechanism to facilitate graduate nurses' role transition. *Journal for Nurses in Staff Development, 24*(2), 49–52.

Thompson, G. (2005). Clinical exemplar. The concept of presencing in perioperative nursing. *AORN Journal, 82*(3), 465. doi:10.1016/S0001-2092(06)60343-8

Waldo, N., & Hermanns, M. (2009). Journaling unlocks fears in clinical practice. *RN, 72*(5), 26–31.

Washington, G. (2009). *Effects of anxiety reducing interventions on performance anxiety in graduate nurses* (Dissertation). Retrieved from http://search.proquest.com/docview/304879730

Wright, S. (2001). Presence of mind. *Nursing Standard, 15*(42), 22–23.

Zisberg, A., Young, H., Schepp, K., & Zysberg, L. (2007). A concept analysis of routine: Relevance to nursing. *Journal of Advanced Nursing, 57*(4), 442–453. doi:10.1111/j.1365-2648.2007.04103.x

PART IV

Role Development: From Advanced Practitioner and Beyond

CHAPTER 17

Networking and Professional Development

Think left and think right and think low and think high. Oh, the thinks you can think up if only you try!

—Dr. Seuss

OBJECTIVES

At the end of this chapter the reader will be able to:

- Understand the significance of networking and professional development
- Identify key components of networking
- Describe the importance of professional organizations
- Understand the importance of subscribing to professional journals
- Identify strategies for joining professional practice committees

The journey of being a student, a new nurse, and beyond is fraught with triumphs and challenges, it comes with a serious obligation and the expectation that you will continue to develop and engage in lifelong learning. Throughout this book various strategies to foster your professional and personal success have been highlighted. Networking is another vital component to your professional development, as both a student and a practitioner. Networking is challenging in the beginning, however, as your confidence builds and you expand you circle of peers and colleagues you will have greater opportunities to network. Networking often involves a quid pro quid approach in which colleagues support each other in their endeavors. Throughout your career you will most likely develop other networks with other professionals who share your passions. For example, if you are a critical care nurse one of your networks might be the American Association of Critical-Care Nurses (AACN). The professionals you network with can help to open doors and provide you with opportunities you would not otherwise be privy to. Learning how to network takes time; however, it is well worth the effort.

THE ART OF NETWORKING

Networking is the process of engaging and communicating with individuals who share similar professions, goals, passions, or other qualities. Typically, this applies to the cultivation of relationships that pertain to business or employment. Networking is related to problem solving, motivation, learning, and access to resources (Taylor, 2013). Taylor (2013) described human capital and social networks in regard to the benefits realized by an organization. "Interestingly the World Health Organization (WHO) (1998) defines networks as: 'A grouping of individuals, organizations and agencies organized on a non-hierarchical basis around common issues or concerns, which are pursued proactively and systematically, based on commitment and trust'" (Taylor, 2013, p. 35.) Networks may consist of small groups or large groups. They may be limited to an organization or a group of organizations that share similar visions. For example, you may network with fellow pediatric nurses in your organization or the entire membership of a professional organization for pediatric nurses. Networking can be particularly helpful when searching for a position as a recommendation from a colleague is a very good endorsement. Networking can be used to help nurses to "enhance career development and professional practice, influence policy and practice, enhance career development and progression, and promote evidence-based practice" (Taylor, 2013, p. 38).

Networking can be accomplished in many different ways—face to face, via the phone, via social media, via snail mail, in addition to various other technologies such as web chatting, blogs, and wikis. Manthey (2010) described the process of using a salon to provide nurses with an opportunity to join together to communicate in small groups. "The word 'salon' comes from France and means intelligent people gathering to talk about important subjects" (Manthey, 2010, p. 232). These informal yet professional meetings usually occur in small groups and may take place in someone's home. Although they may be informal the discussions are serious and include topics such as self-care, reflection, issues and challenges related to the working environment, as well as many other issues. These salons provide a safe, intimate environment for nurses to share both positive and negative experiences. Participants may choose to share an error or an ethical dilemma, the uncertainty of changing one's position, or ambivalence about returning to school. The size and setting of these types of venues foster healing, collegiality, mutual support, and respect. According to Manthey (2012) the salons have been held in Canada and the United States and have grown mostly through word of mouth and web-based invitations.

Networking and mentorship are directly related to professional development in nurses. Furthermore networking is related to career success and leadership development, and is viewed as a means to enhance the nursing profession and its influence on health care. Four types of networks include professional networks, informal networks, organizational membership, and core discussion groups (Nicholl & Tracey, 2007). "Networking has long been considered crucial to successful career development because it provides opportunities for information exchange and collaboration and for career planning and strategy making" (Nicholl & Tracey, 2007, p. 27). Networking involves a reciprocal exchange of knowledge and ideas and provides nurses with access to information, mentors and role models, new trends, and guidance regarding career paths (Scott, 2007).

Technology has expanded the networking circle, which these days can be almost anywhere in the world. For example, social media sites such as Facebook and Twitter provide individuals with the ability to network with various populations in a wide array of geographic locations. For example, Stewart et al. (2012) described the benefits of an international e-networking social media event with nurse midwives. Four countries, New Zealand, Canada, England, and Australia, designed the virtual event. The purpose of this networking event was to share information and knowledge and provide educational material. Another purpose was to share evidenced-based research and to create an international network. Participants were able to interact with world leaders and have access to free educational material (Stewart et al., 2012).

Although Stewart and colleagues do not feel this type of networking should replace face-to-face meetings—based on issues related to time, travel, and the economy—this offers a viable and practical alternative, providing nurses with the multiple benefits of professional networking. One limitation is that Internet access is required, which may prevent some nurses from participating.

Social networking has been widely embraced by many individuals as a means of personal and professional networking. Social media has positive and negative aspects and one must be cautious when using web-based technologies. Tilman Harris (2014) described some of the benefits and concerns of using social networking. The positive aspects include dissemination of educational materials for patients, communication with colleagues, and sharing and disseminating research. Concerns include inappropriate sharing of information and breaches of confidentiality and Health Insurance Portability and Accountability Act (HIPAA) laws. Social networks do provide a venue for networking, however, one must be cognizant of the legal, ethical, and moral issues that govern one's behavior on a social network. It is important to always be professional, remaining aware of the fact that virtually everything you write on a social or web-based program leaves an indelible footprint and cannot be deleted. Guidelines and recommendations for using social media are discussed in greater detail in Chapter 2.

Developing and engaging in networking and joining networks requires you to leave your comfort zone and reach out to various individuals and groups. It is helpful to initially seek networking opportunities in the organizations to which you already belong. For example, as a student you might join a study group or social club. When you begin your new position you will have an opportunity to network with nurses and other members of the health care team. Scott (2007) suggests informal networking may take place in the cafeteria and recommends having an introductory sentence or two prepared for when you meet new colleagues.

A word about business cards: Business cards are an important yet often overlooked tool for new nurses. Business cards can be created on your home computer or purchased for a nominal fee. You should also remember to ask others for their business cards. It is helpful to create a list of the contact information of individuals with whom you would like to network.

You may also consider social media, however, be mindful of its potential dangers and pitfalls. Scott (2007) posits that the biggest mistake one can make is to avoid networking as it provides you with multiple benefits. Networking requires you to take a proactive approach and actively seek out opportunities. Although you may be invited to join a network there is no guarantee you will be accepted, so be sure to join at least one or two networks. You might join one network to discuss career paths and another one to discuss challenges faced as a new nurse. Of course, you do not have to join separate groups to discuss these issues; however, you do want to be sure the networking groups you join are going to meet your needs.

Some networks have been designed to specifically address the needs of student nurses. For example, Oxtoby (2013) described the International Council of Nurses (ICN) student network, which was developed to enable students to network on a global level to discuss issues that specifically pertain to their roles. Additional aims include promoting scientific and extracurricular exchanges, linking nursing students with international health organizations, and recognizing nursing students' responsibility in promoting social justice around the world. Attending the biannual International Council of Nursing conference as a student is a life-changing experience and offers students an opportunity to network on many levels. Even if you are not able to attend, joining this prestigious group will provide you with multiple opportunities to network especially with the ever-expanding and far-reaching capability of the World Wide Web. Being able to communicate and network with student nurses from around the globe and share experiences is really incredible. This is especially helpful for students and nurses who are interested in working or visiting other countries. Learning about how nursing is the same or different in other countries is another benefit of belonging to an international network. Washer (2002) described the benefits of networking using computer-mediated communication with the use of e-mail lists, newsgroups, and chat rooms. Networking can be accomplished in different venues and is extremely beneficial as you transition into your profession and continue on your personal and professional journey.

NETWORKING AND ORGANIZATIONAL MEMBERSHIPS

There are many organizations—professional, formal, and informal— and committees that you can join that will offer you the opportunity to network with a group of like-minded professionals. Guha (2006) posits that scholarly organizations share knowledge and research with their members. Professional organizations include the various nursing associations and offer myriad opportunities for their members. Membership in a professional organization provides opportunities for continuing education, networking, certification, career assistance, and members-only websites (Greggs-McQuilkin, 2005). Some examples of professional organizations include the American Nurses Association, the International Council of Nurses, the American Association of Critical Care Nurses, the National Student Nurses Association, and the Hispanic Nurses Association, just to name a few. There is an association for practically every specialty so you should do some investigating and join one or two professional organizations that relate to your interests or specialty. Membership fees are required in most professional organizations so it may not be feasible to join more than one or two organizations; however, some offer student rates so be sure to ask about reduced rates. Professional organizations hold meetings throughout the year. Some hold one big meeting per year, but have smaller local chapters that hold monthly meetings. Kaweckyj (2009) states, "There are two steps to successful networking: finding people with whom to mingle and then using that time efficiently and productively to your advantage" (p. 14). Attending professional meetings provides you with an opportunity to meet other professionals, however, you need to be proactive and be sure to communicate and exchange contact information with at least a few individuals at the meeting; and don't forget your business cards.

Sigma Theta Tau International Honor Society of Nursing is another organization that is global and offers members many benefits in addition to networking. There are local chapters all over the world and meetings are held at different times each year. Because it is an honor society you are invited to join as a student. It is truly an honor to be invited so do not pass up the opportunity. There is a grade point average (GPA) requirement so if you are interested you should speak with your advisor or faculty representative to see what you can do to strengthen your chances of being selected. If you are not invited as an undergraduate you may be invited when you attend your graduate school program. Sigma Theta Tau also has categories for nursing leaders so if you are not invited to join as a student you may meet the qualifications after you gain some experience as a nursing leader.

There are many other professional groups such as health care groups, advocacy groups, and alumni associations from your college or university. These groups also provide you with an opportunity to network. Hawkins-Dady (2011) described a network forum where different levels of school nurses meet to discuss various issues and have found it to be quite beneficial. There are many opportunities to join various networks and advocacies and you can learn more about this through word of mouth and by searching the Internet. Just be sure to join a reputable organization.

Another great way to network is to volunteer to serve on a committee or task force at your place of employment. Most health care organizations have various committees—some are interprofessional and some are comprised only of nurses. For example, nursing committees include the Nursing Practice Council and the Nursing Research Council. Interprofessional committees include the Safety Committee or

Pharmaceuticals and Therapeutics Committee. If you are interested in a future leadership position you might volunteer to chair one of these committees. These are just a couple of examples, and each organization is unique. Committee membership is a great way to network with your colleagues in nursing and other disciplines. You can also add this to your résumé and it may help you to secure a future position either in another specialty or as a future nursing leader.

Journal clubs are another way to network and you might spearhead the development of one of these committees. Journal clubs most often involve the reading and discussion of current literature, for example, evidence-based practice. In this type of club the chair or leader selects an article and develops some questions for the group to reflect on and discuss at an in-person meeting. Another option would be to develop a group using social media so you could network with individuals from different geographic locations. This is a fun way to network and learn about current research.

Another type of journal club would be related to the art of journaling. This type of club could be held in your organization or via a social media venue. A chair or leader is necessary to arrange meetings and topics. For example, a student topic might be related to the final semester of nursing school with students journaling about their experience and coming together to share and reflect on the major themes—both the challenges and the triumphs.

Social clubs can be formed for any number of reasons and are another way to network and share interests or hobbies; for example, a book club in which a group comes together either in person or via social media to discuss a particular book. The book could be a work of fiction or something that relates to the nursing profession. Again, this is a way to learn, network, and engage in self-care. You might create a gardening club, an art club, or a support group. The possibilities are endless and the benefits are enormous. The meeting dates and times are flexible and may provide an opportunity to focus on something other than your position, which at times can be very stressful. Civic groups are another option and are often voluntary in nature. These groups provide you with an opportunity to network with individuals from various professions and can help you to understand how others view health care. You can learn valuable lessons from these groups and you never know what opportunities will arise from this type of committee. For example, if you are interested in the political arena this can be a great way to learn more about the legislative process. You can also learn how to better advocate for health care and the nursing profession.

CONFERENCES AND PROFESSIONAL JOURNALS

Attending a conference is a great way to network and many of the professional organizations hold at least one conference per year. Conferences usually have a large number of attendees so you will have many opportunities to network. There is often a reduced rate for members and an early-bird special, however, often you do not need to be a member to attend the conference. Conferences are also important for your professional development and your employer may provide financial assistance to offset some of the costs associated with attending.

Journal articles may provide a reader the opportunity to network with the author as many authors include their contact information in the article (Washer, 2002). Even if the author's contact information is not included you can always contact the editor and let him or her know why you wish to contact the author of a particular article.

In summary, networking is extremely important for you on a personal and professional level. There are many places and opportunities to network, however, you need to be proactive and actively seek opportunities for networking. Although you may be more comfortable networking with nurses and peers it is also good to network with other professionals in health care, business, and government.

NETWORKING ETIQUETTE

Networking is an important component of your professional and personal development and you want to be sure to always present yourself in the most professional manner. Wheatman (2011) offers some helpful advice when networking. When talking face to face or via the telephone conduct yourself in a professional manner, communicate effectively, and stay engaged. For example, do not text or check your messages, do not chew gum, and do not interrupt others when speaking. Try to avoid being argumentative and never bad mouth your employer or colleagues. You also need to be reliable and attend scheduled meetings in a timely manner, be prepared for the meeting and complete any tasks in a timely fashion. Business cards are a must and should be professional and up to date. Remember to send thank-you notes to individuals in your network who have offered their assistance or have inspired you in some way. You want to make a good impression as networking may offer you opportunities to advance your career.

TOP 10 TIPS FOR NETWORKING

1. Be proactive in seeking networking opportunities.

2. Be professional in all of your communications.

3. Join a professional organization.

4. Volunteer to chair a meeting.

5. Share business cards.

6. Consider an online networking group.

7. Be dependable and punctual.

8. Join a social or civic group.

9. Engage in a give-and-take relationship.

10. Stay active in your networking groups.

SUMMARY

This chapter focused on the importance of networking for professional development, information sharing, self-care, and the opportunity to engage with others in regard to multiple issues. Strategies for networking were discussed in addition to the benefits of potential membership in a wide variety of professional, social, and civic groups. The importance of networking etiquette was also emphasized.

DISCUSSION QUESTIONS

1. What is the definition of networking?

2. Why should one engage in networking?

3. What are some benefits of networking?

4. What are the benefits of joining a professional organization?

5. List and describe at least three ways to network.

6. What are ways you can ensure network etiquette?

7. What is the definition of a network according to the WHO?

8. What venues can you use to network?

9. What is the benefit of chairing a committee?

10. How can subscribing to a professional journal provide you with an opportunity to network?

SUGGESTED LEARNING ACTIVITIES

- Select one professional organization to join and one professional journal to subscribe to.
- Interview a nurse and a nursing leader about the art of networking.
- Explore networking opportunities via social media.
- Start a journal club at your school or organization.

REFERENCES

Greggs-McQuilkin, D. (2005). Why join a professional nursing organization? *Nursing, 35,* 19.

Guha, M. (2006). The function of the scholarly organization: What is the Royal Society for? *Journal of Mental Health, 15*(5), 513–515.

Hawkins-Dady, H. (2011). Connecting practitioners: A look at a regional networking forum. *British Journal of School Nursing, 6*(2), 63.

Kaweckyj, N. (2009). Networking within your professional association. *Dental Assistant, 78*(5), 12.

Manthey, M. (2010). A talk for all times. *Nursing Forum, 45*(4), 232–236. doi:10.1111/j.1744-6198.2010.00193.x

Nicholl, H., & Tracey, C. (2007). Applied leadership. Networking for nurses. *Nursing Management—UK, 13*(9), 26–29.

Oxtoby, K. (2013). Worldwide student network identifies emerging trends. *Nursing Standard, 27*(35), 64.

Scott, D. (2007). Networking series, Part I: Networking fundamentals for nurses. *Tennessee Nurse, 70*(4), 24–25.

Sigma Theta Tau International Honor Society for Nurses. (2014). *Home page.* Retrieved from www.nursingsociety.org/Membership/Pages/default.aspx

Stewart, S. S., Sidebotham, M. M., & Davis, D. D. (2012). International networking: Connecting midwives through social media. *International Nursing Review, 59*(3), 431–434. doi:10.1111/j.1466-7657.2012.00990.x

Taylor, R. (2013). Networking in primary health care: How connections can increase social capital. *Primary Health Care, 23*(10), 34–40.

Tillman Harris, C. (2014). Social networking and nurses. *Missouri State Board of Nursing Newsletter, 16*(1), 20–21.

Washer, P. (2002). Professional issues. Professional networking using computer-mediated communication. *British Journal of Nursing, 11*(18), 1215–1218.

Wheatman, D. (2011). Five keys to networking etiquette for your career. *Glassdoor Blog.* Retrieved at https://*www.glassdoor.com/blog/keys-networking-etiquette-career/*

World Health Organization (1998). *Health promotion glossary.* Geneva, Switzerland: Author.

CHAPTER 18

Understanding Various Health Care Agencies/Accrediting Bodies

Teamwork is the ability to work together toward a common vision. The ability to direct individual accomplishments toward organizational objectives. It is the fuel that allows common people to attain uncommon results.

—Andrew Carnegie

OBJECTIVES

At the end of this chapter the reader will be able to:

- Understand how regulatory and licensing agencies inform professional practice
- Discuss the role and function of The Joint Commission
- Identify key aspects of the many professional agencies that inform health care and nursing practice

All students and nurses should be knowledgeable about the organizations that are at the forefront of nursing and health care. There are multiple agencies that inform professional practice and serve to guide health care organizations in the delivery of care. Some agencies have a specific role and function, such as the Centers for Disease Control, whereas others are broad in scope, such as The Joint Commission. Oftentimes these agencies work in concert with each other but at times their requirements may be at odds with one another. Your hospital administrators are responsible for interpreting standards and developing policies, procedures, and education to meet these standards. However, you need to be knowledgeable about the standards and how they inform your practice.

These agencies also contain a wealth of information on their websites and in their manuals, and it is helpful to review this information periodically so you have current information. Licensing agencies are the highest authority and health care organizations must be in compliance with all the agencies' regulations and standards in order to continue to operate. The role of the accrediting agencies is to set guidelines for hospitals to deliver a high level of safe and effective quality care. There are myriad professional organizations and, as previously discussed, you should plan to join at least one or two that relate to your specialty or area of interest. It is critical for professions to have professional organizations to generate ideas, knowledge, and energy in advancing the profession and expanding the knowledge base of the discipline (Matthews, 2012). "There are over a hundred national nursing associations and many other international organizations. The website, Nursing Organization Links (NOL, 2011), maintains a web-based list of organizations, yet acknowledges this list is not complete" (Matthews, 2012, para. 7).

LICENSING AGENCIES

In the United States, the highest authority in the oversight of health care organizations resides in the individual states' licensing boards. Other countries have similar regulatory boards. The process for obtaining and maintaining licensure is complex and regulatory agencies work in concert with accrediting agencies.

> For acute care hospitals to operate, regardless of the sponsorship model, they must hold a valid state license. Licensing, a form of state police power, has existed widely since the 1950s and details a set of baseline structural and operational requirements by which hospitals can be surveyed and evaluated. (Blum, 2010, p. 37)

Licensed agencies must also be governed by a board of directors, which follows a set of bylaws. Hospitals that treat patients on Medicare must also comply with the standards set forth by the Medicare Conditions of Participation and The Joint Commission (Blum, 2010). Medicare is a federal program; hence hospitals must comply with state and federal regulations. Medicare Conditions of Participation include the following requirements of a hospital's board of directors (Blum, 2010):

- Appointing a CEO (chief executive officer)
- Credentialing of practitioners
- Ensuring effective patient care
- Developing a budget
- Overseeing contracted health care services
- Maintaining emergency services

Health care organizations have an obligation to provide safe and effective quality of care to all their patients. They also need to ensure that their employees have a safe place in which to practice. It is important for all nurses to understand the process, bylaws, and standards that their organizations are required to follow and to be sure that they are in compliance with these regulations. Some nurses and other employees fail to realize the serious responsibility they have in helping their organizations be compliant with laws and standards of care and practice.

THE JOINT COMMISSION

The Joint Commission (TJC) is an accrediting agency in the United States that is an independent organization founded in 1951 (TJC 1951). "The Joint Commission accredits and certifies more than 20,000 health care organizations and programs in the United States. Joint Commission accreditation and certification is recognized nationwide as a symbol of quality that reflects an organization's commitment to meeting certain performance standards" (TJC, 2014). The Joint Commission has standards for the various types of organizations and conducts accreditation surveys every 3 years. According to The Joint Commission (2014). accreditation has many benefits for an organization. For example, it can help an organization to improve patient outcomes and safety, improve quality of care, and promote a culture of excellence.

All employees are expected to be knowledgeable about The Joint Commission and do their best to comply with its standards. When The Joint Commission comes to survey your organization they spend several days evaluating the organization. They meet with various administrators, employees, and patients. They evaluate practice and compliance to standards, and review medical records and interview patients. They ask employees different types of questions. For example, they may ask you about fire safety or infection control. They might ask you about pain management and then review one of your medical records to see if you addressed and treated pain in accordance with hospital policy. Or they may ask you about patient education and then interview your patient to see what you taught them. Although you may be nervous you just need to be truthful and share what you do on a daily basis. Many hospitals run mock surveys so that employees will be prepared and not overly anxious. The accreditation process should serve as a learning experience and the goal of everyone is to ensure positive patient outcomes.

Although The Joint Commission is a well-known accrediting body in the United States, DiCecco (2010) described another accrediting body, DNV Healthcare; Inc. (DNVHC), which is the accrediting body of Det Norske Veritas (DNV) established in 1864 in Norway. The DNVHC is an international accrediting agency that was granted "deeming authority" in 2008 to survey organizations in the United States that meet or exceed the Medicare Conditions of Participation (CoPs) (DiCecco, 2010, p. 22).

THE DEPARTMENT OF HEALTH

The United States Department of Health and Human Services is an agency run by the federal government. The main purpose of this agency is to provide Americans with access to high-quality health care and help them to live healthy lives. They also assist people in securing jobs and finding affordable child care and promote food safety and best outcomes in health care.

Every country and province has an agency that oversees the health of its citizens. According to the U.K. Department of Health (2014):

> The Department of Health (DOH) helps people to live better for longer. We lead, shape and fund health and care in the UK, making sure people have the support, care and treatment they need, with the compassion, respect and dignity they deserve. (para. 1)

India has the Ministry of Health and Family Welfare, and according to their website:

> Directorate General of Health Services (DGHS) is attached to the office of the Department of Health & Family Welfare and has subordinate offices spread all over the country. The DGHS renders technical advice on all medical and public health matters and is involved in the implementation of various health services. (Ministry of Health and Family Welfare, 2014)

You should become familiar with the mission, vision, and resources of your country's or province's health department. Many of these organizations have valuable resources for patients, families, and nurses.

THE WORLD HEALTH ORGANIZATION

The World Health Organization (WHO) plays an important role in global health. The definition of "health" according to the World Health Organization is "a state of complete physical, mental and social well-being and not merely the absence of disease or infirmity" (WHO, 2014).

The WHO provides leadership on global health issues and monitors health trends and provides technical support to countries. It also plays a role in research and evidenced-based practice (WHO, 1948).

The World Health Organization offers wonderful resources on its website. In today's world international travel is commonplace and potential exposure to certain diseases has risen. It is important for nurses and other health care workers to understand the significance of global health.

CENTERS FOR DISEASE CONTROL AND PREVENTION

The Centers for Disease Control and Prevention (CDC) is an agency based in the United States whose mission is to protect all Americans from health and safety threats at home or abroad. According to the CDC website (CDC, 2014), this agency is responsible for monitoring the health of our nation 24/7 and its role is:

- Detecting and responding to new and emerging health threats
- Tackling the biggest health problems causing death and disability for Americans
- Putting science and advanced technology into action to prevent disease
- Promoting healthy and safe behaviors, communities and environment
- Developing leaders and training the public health workforce, including disease detectives

With the instability throughout our world, now more than ever we need to be prepared for natural and man-made threats to our health and safety. Due to international travel diseases are spread very quickly. Individuals in other countries are more susceptible to certain diseases as they have not been previously exposed and therefore have not developed immunity. Recently, the United States has had outbreaks of measles, a communicable disease that had been eradicated due to a stringent vaccination program. However, some individuals do not believe in vaccinations and therefore we are now dealing with multiple cases of measles.

Unfortunately, we live in a very unstable time and the threat of a terror attack, either biological or chemical, is always looming overhead. Nurses and other health care workers must be prepared to treat myriad conditions and be prepared for the possibilities of both man-made and natural disasters. In recent years there have been several catastrophic natural disasters and nurses have been at the forefront in providing care to multiple victims.

NATIONAL LEAGUE FOR NURSING

The National League for Nursing (2014) is an organization that is based in Washington, DC, and its purpose is to provide support, research, and resources to nurse educators and leaders in nursing education. If you attend nursing school in the United States your nursing program will be accredited by ACEN (Accreditation Commission for Education in Nursing), the accrediting body of the National League for Nursing (NLN), or by the CCNE (Commission on Collegiate Nursing Education), the accrediting body of the American Association of Colleges of Nursing (AACN). These organizations are focused on maintaining excellence in the education and preparation of new nurses. The National League for Nursing includes diploma, associate degree, and baccalaureate programs in their mission. The NLN (2014) subscribes to the following four core values: caring (health promotion), integrity (respecting every person), diversity (affirming differences), and excellence (implementing transformative strategies).

The NLN is a driving force in nursing and is a strong advocate of the profession. It offers a variety of resources and one can join as an organizational or individual member. They also offer various testing services and you may be required to take one of their exams. For example, as part of your application for employment you will be required to pass a medication administration exam, and many organizations use the NLN's medication administration exam because it is a well-developed exam that is reliable and valid.

AMERICAN ASSOCIATION OF COLLEGES OF NURSING

The American Association of Colleges of Nursing (AACN) is similar to the National League for Nursing, however, they provide resources and services only to baccalaureate and graduate programs in nursing. The

American Association of Colleges of Nursing (AACN, 2014) provides resources, leadership, research, and support to member schools with the overarching goal of serving the public interest in regards to nursing and health care. According to the AACN (2014), they embrace the following core values:

- Respecting and including diversity of opinion, experience, and culture
- Open and responsive communication
- Quality, efficiency, and accountability in the implementation and evaluation of activities
- Positioning through integrity

The AACN has the following vision: "By 2020, highly-educated and diverse nursing professionals will lead the delivery of quality health care and the generation of new knowledge to improve health and the delivery of care services" (AACN, 2014, para. 1). Now more than ever nurses must be prepared to practice in a complex setting and possess the knowledge, skills, and critical-thinking ability required to care for diverse complex patients across the life span. Whether your program is accredited by the CCNE or ACEN you should be knowledgeable about the standards that inform your program. You also want to take advantage of resources available to you in the form of literature, conferences, and scholarships for graduate school.

AMERICAN NURSES ASSOCIATION

The American Nurses Association (ANA) was created in 1896 to organize a national association for professional nurses. The American Nurses Association represents the interests of the 3.1 million nurses in the United States and oversees and collaborates with the various state nurses association across the country.

> The ANA advances the nursing profession by fostering high standards of nursing practice, promoting the rights of nurses in the workplace, projecting a positive and realistic view of nursing, and by lobbying the Congress and regulatory agencies on health care issues affecting nurses and the public. (ANA, 2014)

The ANA is a driving force in nursing and represents nurses all around the country. The state associations also function in the capacity of a collective bargaining agency and if your organization is a member you will be required to join your local association. Some health care organizations are unionized and some are not. If your organization is unionized you must join because they represent the collective and individual needs of nurses. On the other hand if your organization is not unionized, although your membership is not mandatory, you may still join as there are many resources available to members. You can learn more about the ANA by visiting its website. Some of the information is restricted to members; however, you will have access to information about the services and resources they provide. According to "Updated Information on the Value of Nurses in the Healthcare Delivery System" (2013), nurses should become actively engaged in their professional organizations so they can help advance health care and the nursing profession.

INTERNATIONAL COUNCIL OF NURSES

The International Council of Nurses (ICN) is a worldwide organization that represents the interests of more than 16 million nurses around the world. The ICN is an international federation that is comprised of 130 nursing associations. It was originally founded in 1899 and its goal is to advance nursing knowledge, develop global health policies, and promote quality nursing care (ICN, 2014).

This is an organization that connects nurses around the world and addresses nursing and health care on a global level. Every 2 years they hold a large conference and students and nurses from all specialties and countries come together to share knowledge and research findings. It is an incredible experience and one that every nurse should attend at least once.

The following is an excerpt written about my experience as a presenter at the International Council of Nurses conference in Malta in 2011:

> It is the supreme art of the teacher to awaken joy in creative expression and knowledge.—*Albert Einstein*

This past May I had the honor of presenting at The International Council of Nurses Conference. The International Council of Nurses (ICN) was founded in 1899 and since that time has grown into a federation consisting of 130 national nurses associations from around the world. The ICN works on an international level to advance the profession of nursing through the development of global policies, the advancement of nursing science, and the provision of quality nursing care (ICN, 2014). From the moment our abstract was accepted I eagerly anticipated this opportunity. Not only was I going to be attending an international conference but I was also going to be presenting with my esteemed colleagues: Dr. Connie Vance (College of New Rochelle professor) and Dr. Launette Woolforde (Corporate Director of Nursing). Then we received the good news that Dr. Taylor (Russel & Deborah Taylor Foundation), was creating a scholarship to support two nursing students to attend the conference.

When reflecting on my participation at the ICN conference the above quote by Albert Einstein captures the very essence of this experience. For this is what I experienced both personally and professionally, and observed on multiple levels while attending this conference. This experience was profound, changed my worldview of nursing, and awakened in me a greater interest in global nursing. It was such a joy to share this journey with colleagues and students from The College of New Rochelle, along with the many nurses that I was privileged to meet. I am also grateful for the generous support I received from The College of New Rochelle to attend this conference. I believe every nurse should attend at least one international conference either as a participant, presenter, or both.

Some of the highlights of the conference were:

- Attending a welcome reception with our nursing leaders from the American Nurses Association
- Meeting Dr. Jean Watson, who spoke so highly of The College of New Rochelle
- Attending the opening-night ceremony, which was like being at the opening ceremony of the Olympics
- Attending a preconference with our colleagues from the University of Alberta to share our scholarly work and discuss future collaborations
- Listening to Dr. Diana Mason's keynote address, along with those of the many other esteemed presenters
- Meeting and learning from a plethora of international researchers and scholars
- Presenting our work on The First Career Stage in Nursing: A Critical Link to the Future of Professional Nursing Practice
- Being in the presence of wonderful nurse colleagues from around the world
- Being welcomed by the Maltese nurses and learning about their history
- Having an opportunity to share a scholarly journey with students and colleagues in the beautiful setting of Malta

SUMMARY

This chapter focused on the various agencies that regulate and support nursing and health care in the United States and around the world. An overview of regulatory, accrediting, government, and professional organizations that inform health care and nursing was provided. The importance of being knowledgeable about the various organizations and the resources available was also discussed, in addition to the requirement that all nurses take an active role in one or more of these organizations.

DISCUSSION QUESTIONS

1. What is the role and function of regulatory agencies?
2. What is the role and function of accrediting agencies?
3. Discuss the role of The Joint Commission.
4. What is the role of the Centers for Disease Control and Prevention?
5. Discuss the role of the American Nurses Association and its history.
6. What is the role and function of the Department of Health?
7. Why is the International Council of Nurses important to all nurses?
8. Describe the role of the National League for Nursing.
9. Describe the role of the American Association of Colleges of Nurses.
10. What is the role and function of the World Health Organization?

SUGGESTED LEARNING ACTIVITIES

- Explore websites of the various agencies.
- Learn about the American Nurses Association.
- Investigate your state's chapter of the American Nurses Association.
- Interview your nursing manager/administrator about the accreditation process.
- Interview two staff nurses about their knowledge of the CDC and ICN.

REFERENCES

American Association of Colleges of Nursing. (2014). *2014 federal policy agenda: Advancing higher education in nursing.* Retrieved from http://www.aacn. nche.edu/government-affairs/AACN_FedPolicy14.pdf

American Nurses Association. (2014). *About ANA.* Retrieved at https://www .ana.org

Blum, J. (2010). The quagmire of hospital governance: Finding mission in a revised licensure model. *Journal of Legal Medicine, 31*(1), 35-57. doi:10.1080/01947641003598229

Centers for Disease Control. (2014). *Home page.* Retrieved at https://www .cdc.gov

DiCecco, K. (2010). A global influence in hospital accreditation. *Journal of Legal Nurse Consulting, 21*(3), 22–24.

The International Council of Nurses. (2014). *Our mission, strategic intent, core values and priorities.* Retrieved at https://www.icn.org

The Joint Commission. (2014). *Facts about The Joint Commission.* Retrieved from https://www.thejointcommission.com.

Matthews, J. H. (2012). Role of professional organizations in advocating for the nursing profession. *Online Journal of Issues in Nursing, 17*(1), 1. doi:10.3912/ OJIN.Vol17No01Man03

The Ministry of Health and Family Welfare. (2014). *Brief history.* Retrieved from http://mohfw.nic.in

National League for Nursing. (2014). *About the NLN: Welcome to the National League of Nursing.* Retrieved at https://www.nln.org/

The U.K. Department of Health. (2014). *What we do.* Retrieved from https:// www.gov.uk/government/organisations/department-of-health

The United States Department of Health and Human Services. (2014). *About HHS.* Retrieved from https://www.hhs.gov

Updated information on the value of nurses in the healthcare delivery system and what nurses can do to spread the great news! (2013). *South Carolina Nurse, 20*(2), 1–11.

World Health Organization. (1948). *Preamble to the constitution of the World Health Organization* (Official Records of the World Health Organization, no. 2, p. 100). Retrieved from http://www.who.int/about/definition/en/ print.html

World Health Organization. (2014). *About WHO.* Retrieved from https://www .who.org.

CHAPTER 19

Future Roles, Advanced Education, Advanced Practice Certifications, and Continuing Education

It's never too late to be what you might have been.

—George Eliot

OBJECTIVES

At the end of this chapter the reader will be able to:

- Discuss issues related to continued role development
- Describe the importance of advancing education
- Select a program of study
- Describe different nursing roles and qualifications
- Understand the significance of certification

There are myriad opportunities and career options for a nurse to consider after she or he completes basic nursing education and transitions into her or his first position. The Institute of Medicine's report *The Future of Nursing* (2010) calls for nurses to become lifelong learners and leaders in health care. Increasing the number of nurses with baccalaureate degrees and higher is also at the forefront of this report. Although you may not be thinking past your first position it is never too early to start planning. While it is not mandatory to earn an advanced graduate degree it is certainly recommended and is a requirement for many positions. For example, if you are planning on a role as a nurse practitioner, nursing leader, or nurse educator you will need to go back to school for a graduate degree (master's, nurse practitioner, doctor of nursing practice, doctorate, etc.), in addition to obtaining the required level of experience. It is never too early or too late to return to school to advance your education. Furthermore, in addition to attending formal academic programs you should also attend formal conferences and continue to read the current literature. You should also consider certification in your specialty. These exams are challenging and a certain amount of continuing education credits are needed to maintain certification status.

OVERVIEW OF ROLES AND SPECIALTIES

There is a saying "the world is your oyster" and this is certainly true of the nursing profession. It is common for a nurse's first role to be a staff nurse because in this position you need to continue to build on your foundation and continue to develop skills and achieve competencies. Specialty units vary for new nurses, with a large number beginning their careers in medical–surgical units, and a smaller number going into critical care, operating room, emergency department, mother–baby, and psychiatric nursing. Some nurses have a passion for being a staff nurse and choose to spend their careers on the same unit for most of their careers. These nurses become experts and often fulfill the role of preceptor and mentor.

Major categories of nursing roles fall under leadership/management, education, and clinical nursing. The following is a list of well-known specialty areas in which registered nurses may practice:

Specialty Areas

- Medical–surgical
- Critical care
- Intensive care
- Burn unit
- Emergency department
- Perioperative
- Ambulatory care
- Gastroenterology
- Pediatrics
- Labor and delivery
- Mother–baby
- Psychiatric
- Home health
- Hospice
- Oncology

- Clinics
- Private offices
- Media
- Political arena

Clinical Roles

- Staff nurse
- Clinical nurse specialist
- Nurse practitioner (e.g., family nurse practitioner)
- Nurse midwife
- Nurse anesthetist
- Occupational health nurse
- Case manager
- School nurse
- Community/public health nurse
- Infection control nurse
- Flight nurse
- Military nurse
- Forensic nurse
- Holistic nurse

Nursing Leadership Roles

- Assistant nurse manager
- Nurse manager
- Clinical coordinator
- Administrative nursing supervisor
- Assistant director of nursing
- Clinical director of nursing
- Vice president of nursing
- Chief nursing officer
- Nurse recruiter
- Research nurse

Educator Roles (including service and academia)

- In-service instructor
- Staff development coordinator
- Unit-based educator
- Clinical nurse educator
- Education specialist
- Clinical instructor
- Adjunct faculty

- Assistant, associate, and professor of nursing
- Clinical placement coordinator
- Simulation coordinator

This is not an all-inclusive list, however, one can see the wide and varied opportunities that are available to registered professional nurses. The following section will provide more details pertaining to some of the roles, in addition to the academic and experiential requirements.

Staff nurses work in a variety of areas and as a new nurse you will often begin your career in a medical–surgical unit because these types of units often have the most open positions. Many nurses begin their careers in medical–surgical units and then transfer to a different specialty unit or field of nursing. On the other hand, many nurses spend their entire careers in medical–surgical units and earn their medical–surgical certification. Some nurses are fortunate to be offered an internship or fellowship in the specialty unit of their choice. Although some nurses are still undecided about their long-term plans, others know from the beginning that perioperative or psychiatric nursing is their passion so fellowships are extremely beneficial.

If you desire to work in a different type of unit there are things you can do to increase the chances of transferring into a new area. For example, you need to demonstrate your professionalism and competency in your current area. You should explore what the requirements are for the role or area and then develop a plan on how you will obtain the necessary education and experience. For example, if you are interested in critical care nursing you can enroll in a critical care course. You should also discuss your goals with your nurse manager. You might also volunteer to float to different units and, although your assignment will be modified based on your competency level, you will be cross-trained and get to know the staff and manager of different units. Many hospitals like to "grow their own" and will help you to prepare for a new role.

Leadership/management roles may be middle management or upper management. The role of the nurse manager is pivotal to a nursing unit and its success. The requirements for the role of the nurse manager or higher level nursing administrator include nursing experience with increasing leadership responsibilities and a graduate degree. You can seek opportunities for development such as team leader, charge nurse, assistant manager/coordinator, or committee chair. Attending leadership development conferences is also helpful. As mentioned, many organizations promote from within and will help you to prepare for a future leadership role. Some organizations will offer you a leadership position with the understanding that you will earn your advanced degree in a specified time period. Nurses who are interested in a leadership role will often begin the path as a charge nurse and continue to transition to a more advanced role. A possible leadership journey might begin with the role of assistant manager, and then nurse manager, to clinical director, and eventually to chief nursing officer. Leadership roles can be very fulfilling; however, they also come with many responsibilities and can be overwhelming for some. You may think a role in nursing leadership is your passion and somewhere along the journey decide that this type of role is not for you. You should never stay in a role that is not meeting your professional and personal needs; it really is okay to change your mind, but it must be done in a professional manner.

Some positions require leadership qualities but do not involve leading or supervising others. These positions include case manager, quality-improvement nurse, and occupational health nurse. The role of the case manager is to review patients' medical records and care in regards to diagnosis, care provided, and preparation for discharge. The quality-improvement nurse evaluates compliance with standards of care and practice and policies and procedures. The occupational health nurse collaborates with the licensed health care provider to oversee mandatory requirements for annual physicals, employee illnesses, and illness exposure. According to the Occupational Safety and Health Administration (OSHA, 2014), occupational health nurses (OHNs) are registered nurses who independently observe and assess the workers' health status with respect to job tasks and hazards. Using their specialized experience and education, these registered nurses recognize and prevent health effects from hazardous exposures and treat workers' injuries/illnesses.

The role of clinical nurse specialist (CNS) and clinical midwife specialist (CMS) has been in existence for many years and applies to various roles and specialties. Both of these roles have the ability to positively influence patient care and health care in general (Wickham, 2013). Throughout the years these roles have waxed and waned, especially in times of economic downturn. The development of the clinical nurse specialist requires demonstrated expertise and experience in a particular area, and graduate education, in addition to certification in one's specialty (Wickham, 2013). "The CNS/CMS has many roles, including clinical specialist, advisor, researcher, educator, change agent, collaborator, leader and administrator" (Wickham, 2013, p. 874). A clinical nurse specialist may serve as an expert and mentor to nurses on various units, and may also work closely with new-graduate nurses.

The role of the nurse practitioner (NP) has become increasingly and widely embraced and respected. The Institute of Medicine's report *The Future of Nursing* (2010, p. 2) calls for all nurses to "practice at the full extent of their education and training" (IOM, 2010). Although this applies to all levels of nurses, the role of the nurse practitioner has been fraught with issues regarding scope of care and practice. Today many states are developing and passing legislation to expand the scope of practice of NPs and develop standardized guidelines for collaboration with physicians. Nurse practitioners provide primary and acute care to a variety of patients and can assess, diagnose, and prescribe medications (American Association of Nurse Practitioners, 2014) To become a nurse practitioner you need an advanced degree at the master's or doctoral level. Practice areas for NPs include acute care, primary care, and long-term health settings. "ANPs have been described by the ICN (2008a) as registered nurses who have acquired expert knowledge, complex decision-making skills and clinical competencies for expanded practice; the characteristics of which are shaped by the context and/or country in which they are permitted to practice" (Haider, 2014, p. 68). Unfortunately, there is no uniformity in regard to scope of practice although that is certainly a goal of many practitioners and nursing leaders, in addition to being one of the foci of *The Future of Nursing report* (IOM, 2010). However, the significance and recognition of the important role NPs play in health care cannot be underestimated and many believe that NPs will continue to play a significant role in primary health care. Nurse practitioners work in many different settings, with some in private practice and others in a hospital or community setting. There has been talk about requiring the doctor of nursing practice (DNP) degree for all NPs, however, this has not occurred. This is certainly something you should consider when selecting NP programs as another focus of the IOM's report *The Future of Nursing* is for nurses to achieve higher levels of education. If you do decide to become an NP you will need to figure out your specialty and also consider whether or not you should earn your DNP.

There is also a great need for nurse educators, especially in the academic setting. The requirements for educator roles include knowledge, experience, and education. Nurse educator roles most often require a graduate degree at the master's level and a doctoral degree for faculty who teach in baccalaureate or higher degree program. Associate degree and diploma programs prefer an advanced degree, however, at times they will hire baccalaureate-prepared experienced nurses as clinical instructors in their area of specialty. For example, a nurse with a BSN (bachelor of science in nursing) who has several years of experience on a medical–surgical unit would be a good candidate to serve as a clinical instructor for medical–surgical nursing students (Hunt, 2013).

ROLE DEVELOPMENT IN PROFESSIONAL NURSING PRACTICE

Role development for professional nursing practice includes experience, academic preparation, and certifications. Cleary et al. (2013) described the results of their study on perceptions of career development in new graduates in Singapore. Four factors were identified as impediments to career development: excessive work hours, lack of support, insufficient opportunities, and lack of funding for advancing one's education. Many new nurses breathe a sigh of relief when they complete their basic degrees and enter into professional practice. Some get "shivers down their spine" just thinking about going back to school. However, this should be given serious thought and consideration as it will have a positive impact on your career.

There are many ways to develop your role and although earning an advanced degree is desirable there are other things you need to accomplish. For example, as a new nurse you need to develop a plan for how you will advance through Benner's (1984) stages of novice to expert—time, education and experience are all required to advance to these stages. The most important thing is to set realistic and achievable goals (see Chapter 20). The first step is to master the role that you are currently in by increasing your knowledge, critical-thinking and problem-solving skills, and improving time management and organizational skills, in addition to achieving clinical competence in all areas.

There is an old adage that you should learn something new every day; you should aim to meet that goal. Although you may not be ready to go back for an advanced degree there are many ways to engage in active learning. Attending seminars and continuing-education courses on a consistent basis is required of all nurses. Most health care organizations offer at least a few continuing education courses and may also reimburse you for one or two outside conferences per year. You can also earn continuing-education credits by reading continuing-education articles and completing post-tests in various journals. Furthermore, staying abreast of current literature and research is extremely important, especially with health care changing so rapidly.

As stated, earning an advanced degree is highly advisable and many hospitals and other health care organizations offer generous tuition programs. There are various scholarship programs and many professional organizations also offer scholarships to qualified candidates. Even if you do not have a particular role in mind it is wise to continue your formal and informal education throughout your nursing career. Although we still have three paths—associate degree, diploma, and baccalaureate degree, the landscape is changing in certain geographic locations, with the BSN being considered for entry into practice. Today most advanced practice roles require a master's or doctoral degree. For example, roles in nursing leadership, clinical specialist, advanced practice nurses, and educators require an advanced degree. However, if you have the required experience and are enrolled in a program of study many organizations will offer you a position in leadership or as a clinical instructor. The key is to actively seek out opportunities where you can begin to develop experience in these roles. For example, if you are interested in a teaching role you should volunteer to be a preceptor, join the Patient Education Committee, try to publish a continuing-education article and/or submit an abstract on a topic you are expert in for consideration of an oral or poster presentation.

Earning certification in a specialty area is also a great way to demonstrate your abilities and commitment. Adding these to your résumé will demonstrate your ability and interest in this role. On the other hand if a leadership role is your goal, then seek out opportunities to develop and demonstrate your abilities. Becoming a charge nurse or volunteering to chair a committee or lead a unit-based group are ways to begin to develop your leadership skills in addition to continuing your education. Oftentimes someone recognizes your potential before you do, so if you are invited to serve in a leadership capacity you should give it some serious thought. The key is to find a balance and be realistic as transitioning to a leadership role without the required knowledge and skills can set you up for failure. Leadership roles are not for every nurse, however, they can be very rewarding when you find the right fit. In summary, role development is important for every nurse regardless of position or specialty because in addition to personal and professional gains the more important focus is in your ability to provide patient care that is based on current evidence and research and focuses on safety and positive outcomes.

EDUCATIONAL PROGRAMS AND OPTIONS

There are so many educational programs available to nurses that it can be a daunting experience to select the program that will best meet your needs (Federwisch, 2010). Furthermore, you should allow plenty of time for this process as you will need time to explore programs, consult with your place of employment regarding tuition benefits and scheduling conflicts, complete the application process, and arrange your professional and personal schedule.

The following is a list of degrees related to nursing (this is not all inclusive):

- Bachelor's degree in nursing (BSN) (preferred) or other field
- Master's degree in nursing (MS) (preferred) (various specialties) or other field

- Master's in business administration (MBA)
- Nurse practitioner
- Clinical nurse specialist
- Clinical midwife specialist
- Nurse anesthetist (NA)
- Doctor of nursing practice (DNP) (clinical doctorate)
- Doctor of philosophy (PhD) (research degree)
- Post master's certificate programs in various specialties

Once you decide to return to school, whether for personal or professional reasons, you will need to consider many factors. For example, you will need to decide which program of study you are considering. It is extremely important to select an accredited program, whether it is online or in a traditional setting. Accredited programs are recognized as meeting guidelines and standards in providing a quality education to their students. Online programs offer greater flexibility; however, you need to be organized, motivated, and an independent learner, because it is very easy to fall behind. Online programs are just as challenging, and at times more challenging than traditional programs. Some of you will be returning to school for your bachelor's degree, and therefore it is important to consult with an admissions counselor about transferrable credits from your associate degree or diploma program. Some other factors to consider for all programs of study are "class and clinical schedules, library hours, the location of clinical sites, and parking" (Hunt, 2006, para. 7). You will also want to know what type of support programs are available (for example, programs to help you improve your writing skills). Whether in an online or traditional program, you will need access to a computer and the Internet as many programs require online submissions and communication via e-mail. Juggling a career, family, and school can be very challenging, and although you may be eager to earn your degree attending on a part-time basis may be your best option (Hunt, 2006). You also need to consider the costs related to attending school and/or decreasing work hours to accommodate school schedules. Many organizations do offer tuition reimbursement; however, due to the recent economic downturn some organizations have decreased their tuition-assistance programs. One caveat to keep in mind is that ideally one of your advanced degrees be in nursing. This is especially relevant when considering a nurse educator role. Furthermore, many graduate programs will only admit students who have a bachelor's degree in nursing. Another option to consider is programs that offer a dual degree. Currently there are dual-degree programs for associate and baccalaureate degrees. There are also BSN to DNP programs in which students are admitted and on completion earn an MSN and DNP degree. This is an excellent option when you are certain about your career path and future goals. The most important thing to remember is to explore all of your options and weigh the pros and cons before you select your program. Seeking advice from peers, colleagues, and mentors is also advisable. Try not to wait too long to return to school because the longer you wait the harder it is to get back into the role of a student. In the past there was a requirement for at least 2 years of nursing experience prior to applying for a graduate program. However, in most schools this is no longer necessary.

The application process is usually lengthy and time-consuming and is most often completed online. Every academic program has different requirements, procedures, and deadlines so be sure to carefully review each one. Many graduate schools require a minimum GPA (grade point average; 3–3.3) from your undergraduate program, official transcripts, letters of reference, and a personal essay. If you are applying to a baccalaureate program you will have similar expectations with the exception of the GPA, which may be a bit more flexible. Remember that transcripts and letters of recommendation take time so be sure to apply well in advance of the application deadline. Some programs have rolling admissions so you have more flexibility with deadlines. It is a good idea to start planning at least a year before you hope to begin the program. Some health care organizations offer onsite programs with a cohort of nurses from different units. This is a wonderful option as classes will be held in a convenient location, and you can develop a study group with your colleagues. Furthermore, there is often financial support for onsite programs. As you can see there are many options available and the key is to find the right fit.

A major consideration when returning to school is the financial piece, as financial aid is not an option for graduate degrees. It is to be hoped that your place of employment offers a generous tuition-assistance program, however, in order to be eligible you need to pass the course and in most cases you need to pay first and receive reimbursement after successful completion of the course.

There are other options, too, such as personal loans and scholarship money, although scholarships are competitive. Another option in addition to onsite programs is working in a hospital that is affiliated with a university, which provides you with the option of attending their academic programs for little or no cost. Keep in mind that books are costly and are often not included in tuition-assistance programs. Haag (2013) described how one hospital raised money to help their nurses pay for their tuition and/or certification. The program has been very successful and they have raised over $1 million. Since this program has been so successful perhaps others will follow suit. There are many foundations, such as the Jonas Foundation and the Robert Wood Johnson Foundation, that offer scholarships for advanced degrees, thus you will want to explore all of your options. The benefits of earning an advanced degree are well worth the effort and even if you cannot secure funding you may be able to afford a city or state university program.

CERTIFICATION, CONTINUING EDUCATION PROGRAMS, AND CONFERENCES

Certification in your area of specialty demonstrates a higher level of competence and is related to improved patient outcomes (Williams & Counts, 2013). "The purpose of a nursing certification examination is to evaluate the extent to which patient care providers have attained the knowledge and skills necessary for competent practice in a particular specialty" (Williams & Counts, 2013, p. 197). Certification exams have specific requirements and are usually very challenging and require one to study and prepare. There are usually review books and courses you can take to help you to prepare for these exams. You need to check specific guidelines but you must have at least 2 years of experience before you are eligible to sit for the exam. There are certifications for nearly every specialty and one well-known testing organization is the American Nurse Credentialing Center (ANCC), which is a subsidiary of the American Nurses Association (ANA). They offer a variety of certifications for advanced practice nurses in addition to specialty certification for staff nurses. According to the ANCC website, the following eligibility criteria are needed to sit for the medical–surgical nursing certification:

Eligibility criteria:

- Hold a current, active RN license within a state or territory of the United States or the professional, legally recognized equivalent in another country
- Have practiced the equivalent of 2 years full time as a registered nurse
- Have a minimum of 2,000 hours of clinical practice in the specialty area of medical–surgical nursing within the last 3 years
- Have completed 30 hours of continuing education in medical–surgical nursing within the last 3 years

Once you achieve certification you will need to earn a certain amount of continuing education credits every 3 years and apply for recertification. There are many ways to complete continuing education credits and this should be done regardless of certification. Furthermore, some states and countries require a certain amount of continuing-education credits for relicensure. Some programs require the completion of another exam.

There are other programs that offer certifications; for example, the American Association of Critical Care Nurses offers the Critical Care Registered Nurse (CCRN) certification exam and the National League for Nursing offers the Certified Nurse Educator exam. You can find a wealth of information on the Internet regarding eligibility, preparation, and costs for specialty certifications. Some organizations do offer a small increase in pay when nurses achieve certification in their specialty. They may even pay for you to take a review course for the exam as it is a benefit to patients and the hospital to have a cadre of certified nurses. Although certification is not mandatory it is highly recommended so be sure to consider this as you develop your 5-year plan and beyond.

Attendance at conferences, whether for earning approved continuing-education credits or not, is extremely beneficial for knowledge development, sharing research, and networking. You should plan on attending at least one or two formal conferences or seminars every year. In summary, all nurses have an obligation to their patients and profession to be the best nurses they can be.

Top 10 Tips for Role Development

1. Develop a short-term and long-term plan.
2. Explore different professional roles.
3. Evaluate your current level of education, experience, and skills.
4. Consult with your manager and mentor.
5. Continue your education.
6. Volunteer for committees.
7. Ask to be cross-trained for different areas.
8. Attend conferences.
9. Become certified in a specialty area.
10. When opportunity knocks, open the door.

Summary

This chapter focused on the various roles one can engage in as a registered professional nurse. Several roles were highlighted in regard to scope and required education and experience. The importance of professional role development in regard to continuing your education with formal academic programs of study, reading the literature, attending conferences, becoming certified in a specialty, and completing continuing-education programs was also discussed.

Discussion Questions

1. List and describe three nursing roles.
2. What are the benefits of an advanced degree?
3. List and describe four things you need to consider when selecting a program.
4. Why is it important to attend an accredited program?
5. When should you begin the application process for your advanced degree?
6. What are the benefits of becoming certified?
7. List and describe three ways for you to continue your knowledge development.
8. How can you earn continuing education credits?
9. How many conferences per year should you plan on attending?
10. Why is it so important to continue your formal and informal education?

Suggested Learning Activity

- Explore requirements for certification in an area of interest/specialty.
- Compare and contrast pros and cons of online and traditional academic programs of study.

- Interview a nurse and a nurse manager about their commitment to lifelong learning.
- Complete one continuing-education course online or in person.
- Interview a nurse in a specialty of your interest and be sure to ask her or him about her or his role, educational and experiential requirements, and academic preparation.

REFERENCES

American Association of Critical Care Nursing. (2014). *Certification.* Retrieved from https://www.aacn.org

American Association of Nurse Practitioners. (2014). *All about NPs.* Retrieved from http://www.aanp.org/all-about-nps

American Nurse Credentialing Center. (2014). Retrieved from https://www.ancc.org

Benner, P. (1984). *From novice to expert: Excellence and power in clinical nursing practice.* Menlo Park, CA: Addison-Wesley.

Cleary, M., Horsfall, J., Muthulakshmi, P., Happell, B., & Hunt, G. (2013). Career development: Graduate nurse views. *Journal of Clinical Nursing, 22*(17/18), 2605-2613. doi:10.1111/jocn.12080

Federwisch, A. (2010). It's academic: When it comes to advanced degrees, nurses have myriad educational options. *Nurseweek, 17*(4), 18–19.

Haag, V. (2013). How one hospital helps staff nurses pay for advanced academic degrees. *American Nurse Today, 8*(1), 63–65.

Haidar, E. (2014). The reality of introducing advanced nurse practitioners into practice. *Journal of Community Nursing, 28*(1), 68–72.

Hunt, D. (2006). The second time around. *Nurse.com.* Retrieved from https://www.nurse.com.

Hunt, D. (2013). *The new nurse educator: Mastering academe.* New York, NY: Springer Publishing Company.

The Institute of Medicine. (2010). *The future of nursing report brief.* Retrieved from https://www.iom.edu

National League for Nursing. (2014). *Certification for nurse educators.* Retrieved from http://www.nln.org/certification/

United States Department of Health. (2014). *Occupational Safety & Health Administration.* Retrieved from https://www.osha.gov/

Wickham, S. (2013). What are the roles of clinical nurses and midwife specialists? *British Journal of Nursing, 22*(15), 867-875.

Williams, H. F., & Counts, C. S. (2013). Certification 101: The pathway to excellence. *Nephrology Nursing Journal, 40*(3), 197-253.

CHAPTER 20

Developing Short-Term and Long-Term Goals and Objectives

Do not go where the path may lead go instead where there is no path and leave a trail.

—Ralph Waldo Emerson

OBJECTIVES

At the end of this chapter the reader will be able to:

- Understand goal-setting theory and the theory of goal attainment
- Understand the importance of professional role development
- Understand the difference between short-term and long-term plans
- Describe strategies for meeting goals and challenges.

Professional role development and continued socialization into the profession begins as a student and continues throughout one's career. The development of a short- and long-term plan can help to motivate and guide you along your personal and professional journey. The act of developing the plan with realistic goals and objectives provides you with guidance and the steps to follow to achieve your personal and professional goals. This really does help to keep you focused and on track because time goes by so quickly, especially when working full time, and balancing other areas of your life. The plan you develop should be realistic and because it is your own personal plan you can revise it to meet your current goals. When you first develop your plan you may have a totally different journey in mind; however, many opportunities will come your way and you may need to adjust your plan. The important thing is to know that you control your destiny, remembering that some things are beyond our control.

GOAL-SETTING THEORY AND GOAL ATTAINMENT THEORY

Goal setting theory (Locke & Latham, 1991) is based on 35 years of research by Locke and Latham, who identified the moderators of goal-setting—goal commitment, self-efficacy, feedback, and task complexity. When one achieves one's goals he or she experiences satisfaction, which is also viewed as a factor in achieving one's goals and in turn achieving one's goals influences the continued setting of new goals. Interestingly, the more complex the goal the more likely one is to achieve it. According to Locke and Latham (1991), "Goal-setting theory is fully consistent with social–cognitive theory in that both acknowledge the importance of conscious goals and self-efficacy" (p. 714). You may find this theory useful when developing your personal goals, which should be challenging, yet realistic and attainable.

King (1999) developed a theory of goal attainment that describes the interaction and relationship between patients and nurses in the achievement of patient goals, which is related to quality of care and patient satisfaction. Although King's (1981) theory of goal attainment relates to the interaction between nurses and patients in regard to outcomes, it may have applicability when achieving personal goals, too. For example, interactions with mentors and other influential individuals in your life will help you to achieve your professional goals. King's theory describes a dynamic, interpersonal relationship in which a person grows and develops to attain certain life goals (Nursing Theories, 2012). Bularzik et al. (2013) found a positive relationship between perceptions of nurse autonomy, goal attainment, and high-quality patient outcomes. Furthermore, nurse managers played a key role in creating positive work environments and autonomy among their staff nurses.

There are many theories that influence your role as a nurse and certainly the theory of goal attainment will influence your personal and professional development in addition to your interactions and interpersonal relationships with your patients. Intuitively one must acknowledge the relationship of nurses' personal and professional goal attainment and their ability to assist their patients in achieving goals. King's (1999) model depicts a dynamic process of interaction among personal, interpersonal, and social systems. This is a complex process that requires role perception and an ability to communicate and interact with patients and families within a specific environment (King, 1999).

Using a development program can help you to achieve your goals. For example, O'Loughlin et al. (2005) found a positive relationship between completing a professional development program and continued role socialization in physical therapy students. Similarly, developing a 5-year plan with specific goals and objectives will also lead to continued role development and socialization.

DEVELOPING A PLAN

Developing a plan for your continued role development is certainly not mandatory although it is strongly recommended. Anakwe, Hall, and Schor (1999) posit that career management requires individuals to become lifelong learners, develop networking and mentoring relationships, and take responsibility for their own careers. The 5-year plan is often recommended as it gives enough time to accomplish goals without procrastination. Hamakiotis (2013) recommends that nursing students and nurses develop a 5-year plan for effective career advancement. In their Career Pathways Toolkit, Social Policy Research Associates (SPR, 2001), recommend that the time frame of your plan should relate to your overall goal. The plan should have at least one or two goals with objectives and actions you will take to accomplish the goals and may relate to your academic goals or future roles you hope to attain, or both. These are suggestions, but keep in mind the plan should be unique to your needs and goals, hence you should follow whatever strategies you believe will work best for you. For example, perhaps you will want to build in a small reward or celebration when you achieve certain goals. You might want to develop a daily or weekly checklist or perhaps a 6-month checklist. Meeting with your mentor periodically to review your progress can also be helpful. Experimenting with different approaches can help you to determine the best way for you to accomplish your goals. Everyone has a different journey with some having a very smooth and direct path and others having a windy and rough path. Be that as it may, with persistence, perseverance, and a positive attitude you will eventually reach your goal. Granted, the final destination may be quite different than what you had planned or expected because as we learn and develop we often change our goals.

GOALS AND OBJECTIVES

Developing a plan with a realistic goal and measureable objectives takes time, effort, and knowledge. Following the steps in the nursing process—assessment, planning, interventions, and evaluation—can be most helpful when developing your 5-year plan with short- and long-term goals and objectives. Initially you need to give some thought as to where you would like to be in 5 years and 10 years as this will influence your plan. Assessment should be done to identify your current level of skills and knowledge in relationship to your future plan. The results of this self-evaluation will guide the development of your goals and objectives. Many individuals confuse goals and objectives, which are related but very different. A goal defines something you want to achieve. The goal is always first and is usually a broad statement or two about what you hope to achieve on completion of the plan. The objectives identify the narrow and measurable steps you will need to accomplish to achieve your goals. They are written in clear and concise statements—underneath the objectives are the actions you will take to meet your objectives. Objective statements may be written in the cognitive, affective, or psychomotor domains. Cognitive objectives relate to knowledge development, affective objectives relate to attitudes or feelings, and psychomotor objectives relate to acquisition of skills.

The acronym SMART (specific, measurable, attainable, realistic, and time bound) (Love to Know, 2010, as cited in Lee, 2010), may be helpful when developing goals and objectives. Finding a balance between challenging and realistic goals requires careful planning. If your goals are too easy they may not result in a significant change in your personal and professional development. On the other hand if the goals are too challenging you may become overwhelmed and abandon your plan before you have an opportunity to accomplish something.

EXAMPLE OF A PLAN WITH GOALS AND OBJECTIVES

Plan: To earn an advanced degree
Goal: To graduate with a bachelor's degree by 2020
Objective 1: To enroll in an accredited program by 2016
Actions: Explore five college websites by May 2015
　　　　　　Visit at least three colleges by July 2015

Meet with the HR department by August 2015

Begin application process by September 2015

Evaluation: June 2016: Enrolled in a BSN program

This is just one example of ways to develop a plan with realistic and achievable goals, objectives, and actions. As you near completion of your initial goal you will want to develop a new plan. If you have not achieved your original goal you need to revise your plan with a new set of goals, objectives, and actions. As a new nurse you should be well versed in the nursing process, which will be of tremendous help when developing, evaluating, and revising your plan.

WAYS TO STAY ON TRACK OR GET BACK ON TRACK

There are multiple reasons why a plan may not end up being successful, however, there are strategies you can employ to improve your chances of success. As previously stated developing a realistic, achievable, and measurable plan is the key. Building in small rewards and celebrations will also serve as a motivator. Evaluating and revising your plan based on your current needs and situation is also helpful. Larsen (2011) suggests that when roadblocks occur you need to be flexible and find new routes to achieve your goals. Cooper (2003) described the fear factor in some individuals that prevents them from achieving career goals. He posits that many people stagnate in their careers because they fear a risk of failure. However, if one wants to advance in his or her career he or she has to face the challenge and take a chance. Granted, it may be challenging and you may not achieve the goals you planned, however, it is worth the risk. Remember the old adage, *if at first you don't succeed try and try again.* The key is to evaluate why you didn't achieve your goals and develop a revised plan. Having a good support system via friends, family, mentors, and colleagues is also important as you need cheerleaders to motivate you and celebrate your achievements. There are also professional career counselors who you might consult with in helping you to figure out what you hope to achieve and how to develop a plan to reach your destination. Some colleges/universities/organizations provide this type of service at no cost to their students and/or employees so be sure to take advantage of any programs that avail themselves to you. Some additional strategies you might try are to develop a checklist (daily, weekly, monthly, or yearly) and place a big star or checkmark next to the items you have completed. Or you might want to purchase a big white board or cork board and cover it with motivational quotes and a checklist. You can also schedule meetings with your mentor to discuss your progress or lack thereof. With every small action you complete you will become more motivated as you get closer to reaching your goal. You might even buy a big piece of oak tag and make a game board with your goals, objectives, and actions. Whenever you complete an action you advance your game piece and select a prize. These are just a few suggestions that you might find helpful. If you believe in yourself you will achieve your goals.

Top 10 Tips for Goal Development

1. Complete a self-assessment prior to setting goals.
2. Use the nursing process.
3. Be realistic.
4. Challenge yourself.
5. Develop clear goals.
6. Develop measurable objectives.
7. Develop actions with expected dates of completion.
8. Seek input from mentors.
9. Develop a strategy for staying on track.
10. Reward yourself and celebrate your achievements.

Summary

This chapter focused on goal setting in relation to your personal, professional, and academic journey. Goal-setting theory and the theory of goal attainment were discussed. Strategies for developing a realistic plan were presented and the difference between goals and objectives was explained. Strategies for staying on track with your plan and ways to address challenges were also discussed. A template for a self-assessment and a 5-year plan are included in the Appendix.

Energy and persistence conquer all things.

—Benjamin Franklin

DISCUSSION QUESTIONS

1. Discuss goal-setting theory.
2. Discuss the theory of goal attainment.
3. What is a goal?
4. What is an objective?
5. Compare and contrast goals and objectives.
6. Give an example of a cognitive objective.
7. Give an example of an affective objective.
8. Give an example of a psychomotor objective.
9. List three strategies for achieving your goals.
10. What should you do if you do not meet your goals?

SUGGESTED LEARNING ACTIVITY

- Develop a 5-year plan with short- and long-term goals and objectives.
- Interview a staff nurse, nurse manager, and nurse educator about their career paths.

APPENDIX

SELF-ASSESSMENT OF SKILLS AND COMPETENCIES

Please check and complete all that apply

___Academic degrees: _____

___Clinical experience: _____

    Specialties: _____

___Desired comptencies:_____

_____

_____

_____

___Interpersonal skills

___Self-directed

__Learning style: _____

__Organization and time-management skills: _____

Plan for improvement: _____

__Communication skills: _____

Plan for improvement: _____

__Current certifications: _____

Plan for earning certifications: _____

__Continuing-education credits: _____

__Membership in professional organizations: _____

Career goals: _____

Academic goals: _____

Personal goals: _____

This checklist may be used as a self-assessment and to create a 5-year plan.

TEMPLATE: FIVE-YEAR CAREER PLAN (INCLUDE EDUCATIONAL AND PROFESSIONAL GOALS, MEASURABLE OBJECTIVES, AND A SPECIFIC PLAN)

Long-term goals:	
Objective 1 **Objective 2**	
Plan 1. 2. 3. 4.	**Actions and expected dates of completion:** _____ _____ _____ _____
Short-term goals:	
Objective 1 **Objective 2**	
Plan 1. 2. 3. 4.	**Actions and expected dates of completion:** _____ _____ _____ _____

REFERENCES

Anakwe, U. P., Hall, J. C., & Schor, S. M. (1999). Career management in changing times: Role of self-knowledge, interpersonal knowledge, and environmental knowledge. *Academy Of Management Proceedings & Membership Directory,* C1–C6. doi:10.5465/APBPP.1999.27595494

Bloom, B. S. (1956). *Taxonomy of educational objectives, handbook I: The cognitive domain.* New York, NY: David McKay Co.

Bularzik, A. H., Tullai-McGuinness, S., & Sieloff, C. (2013). Nurses' perceptions of their group goal attainment capability and professional autonomy: A pilot study. *Journal of Nursing Management, 21*(3), 581–590. doi:10.1111/j.1365-2834.2012.01381.x

Cooper, B. (2003). Career coach. What's your "fear factor"? Facing your fears can help you achieve your career goals—And you don't have to walk on glass or take a snake bath. *PT: Magazine of Physical Therapy, 11*(6), 31.

Hamakiotis, M. (2013). Career planning in nursing—Do you have a five-year plan? *Canadian Journal of Neuroscience Nursing, 35*(1), 19.

King, I. M. (1981). A theory for nursing: Systems, concepts, process. Albany, NY: Delmar.

King, I. M. (1999). A theory of goal attainment: philosophical and ethical implications. *Nursing Science Quarterly, 12*(4), 292–296.

Lee, K. (2010). Planning for success: Setting SMART goals for study. *British Journal of Midwifery, 18*(11), 744–746.

Locke, E. A. (1991). Goal theory vs. control theory: Contrasting approaches to understanding work motivation. *Motivation and Emotion, 15,* 9–28.

Locke, E. A., & Latham, G. P. (2002). Building a practically useful theory of goal setting and task motivation: A 35-year odyssey. *American Psychologist, 57*(9), 705–717. doi:10.1037/0003-066X.57.9.705

Love to Know. (2010) *Business. Examples of SMART goals and objectives.* Retrieved from http://business.lovetoknow.com/wiki/Examples_of_ SMART_Goals_and_Objectives

Nursing Theory. (2012). *Imogene King's theory of goal attainment.* Retrieved from http://currentnursing.com/nursing_theory/goal_attainment_theory.html

O'Loughlin, K., Dal Bello-Haas, V., & Milidonis, M. (2005). The professional development plan: Cultivation of professional development and lifelong learning in professional (entry-level) physical therapist students. *Journal of Physical Therapy Education, 19*(2), 42–51.

Social Policy Research Associates. (2011). *Career pathways toolkit: Six key elements for success.* Retrieved from www.workforceinfodb.org/PDF/ CareerPathwaysToolkit2011.pdf.

Index